BLUE ZONE DIET 2024

110 Delicious Recipes Eat to Live, the Path to Longevity, Your Practical Guide to Healthy Living

KLARLOCK

DISCLAIMER

This book aims to provide useful and informative material on the topics covered in the publication. It is sold with the understanding that the author and publisher are not engaged in rendering any personal medical, health care, or other professional services in the book. The reader should consult his or her physician, health care provider, or other competent professional before adopting any suggestions in this book or drawing any conclusions. The author and publisher expressly disclaim responsibility for any liability, loss, or risk, personal or otherwise, arising, directly or indirectly, from the use and application of any contents of this book.

NOTE

In the context of this book, when we refer to "a cup" as a unit of measurement for ingredients, we mean using a standard kitchen cup with a capacity of approximately 2 milliliters. It is essential to use a measuring cup to get the right quantities of ingredients. If you don't have a measuring cup, you can use a graduated measuring cup, making sure to correctly correspond to the proportions indicated. Here are some examples 1 Cup of flour 100 gr. 1 cup of rice 200 gr. 1 Cup of Quinoa 200 g, It is recommended to level the dry ingredients in the cup using a spatula or the blade of a knife to obtain an accurate measurement. For liquid ingredients it is recommended to fill the cup to the brim without squeezing or leaving gaps.

TABLE OF CONTENT

RECIPES SECOND DISHES

INTRODUCTION WELCOME TO THE BLUE ZONE

Welcome to the Blue Zone of 2024. In an age where the pursuit of wellness and longevity has become a priority for many, the Blue Zone diet presents itself as a guiding beacon towards a longer, healthier and happier life. The Blue Zone, a term coined by journalist Dan Buettner, identifies the regions of the world where people live longer and healthier than the rest of the global population. These "Blue Zones" include places like Okinawa in Japan, Ikaria in Greece, and Nicoya in Costa Rica, where longevity is a norm, not an exception. But what makes these regions so special? The answer lies in a combination of factors, including nutrition, lifestyle, genetics and social environment. And nutrition is one of the key elements that distinguish the populations of the Blue Zone.

Over the years, scholars have carefully studied the eating habits of these communities, identifying common patterns that promote longevity and health. Based on the latest scientific discoveries and the expertise of experts in the fields of nutrition and health, this book will provide readers with a complete guide to adopting a Blue Zone-inspired lifestyle, promoting not only greater longevity, but also better life quality. Through a combination of theory and practice, we will explore the fundamental principles of the Blue Zone diet, provide practical advice on how to plan meals, prepare delicious recipes, and stay motivated on the path to health and longevity.

Additionally, we'll examine the multiple health benefits of adopting the Blue Zone lifestyle, from increased energy and vitality to reducing the risk of chronic disease. But the Blue Zone diet goes beyond simple nutrition: it also involves other fundamental aspects of lifestyle, such as physical activity, stress management and social connections. Therefore, throughout the book we will also explore these themes, offering readers a comprehensive and integrated view of how best to embrace the Blue Zone lifestyle in 2024 and beyond. We are excited to share this journey to a healthier, longer, happier life with you. Get ready to explore the secrets of the world's longest-lived populations and transform your life with the 2024 Blue Zone Diet

DISCOVERING THE BLUE ZONE

The Blue Zones are five regions of the world where people live exceptionally long and healthy lives. These regions are: Sardinia, Italy: Sardinia is home to one of the highest rates of centenarians in the world. The longevity of Sardinians is believed to be due to a combination of factors, including their Mediterranean diet, active lifestyle and strong social ties. Sardinia, Italy Okinawa, Japan: Okinawa is a Japanese island known for its high concentration of centenarians. The Okinawan diet is rich in fish, vegetables and legumes and is thought to contribute to their longevity. Nicoya Peninsula, Costa Rica: The Nicoya Peninsula is another region with a high rate of centenarians. Costa Ricans' longevity is believed to be due to a combination of factors, including diet, active lifestyle and low stress level.

Loma Linda, California: Loma Linda is a city in California home to a large community of Seventh-day Adventists. Seventh-day Adventists are known for their healthy lifestyle, which includes a vegetarian diet, regular exercise, and non-smoking. Ikaria, Greece: Ikaria is a Greek island known for its high rate of centenarians. The Ikarians' longevity is believed to be due to a combination of factors, including their Mediterranean diet, active lifestyle and strong social bonds. Researchers have studied the inhabitants of the Blue Zones to try to understand the secrets of their longevity. They found that Blue Zoners share a number of habits that contribute to their health and longevity, including: Diet: Blue Zoners eat a plant-based diet rich in fruits, vegetables, legumes and whole grains. They also eat meat and fish in moderation.

Exercise: Blue Zone residents regularly exercise, often as part of their daily lives. Social Engagement: Blue Zone residents have strong social ties with family and friends. Stress Management: Blue Zoners have healthy ways to manage stress, such as meditation and yoga. Sense of Purpose: Blue Zoners have a strong sense of purpose in life. If you're interested in living a longer, healthier life, you may consider adopting some of the habits of Blue Zoners. Eating a healthy diet, exercising regularly, cultivating strong social relationships, managing stress, and finding a sense of purpose in life can help you live a longer, more fulfilling life.

WHAT IS THE BLUE ZONE

The "Blue Zone" is a term coined by journalist Dan Buettner to identify regions of the world where people live longer and healthier lives than the rest of the global population. These areas include places like Okinawa in Japan, Ikaria in Greece, and Nicoya in Costa Rica, where longevity is the norm, not the exception. Longevity regions, or Blue Zones, are characterized by a number of factors that promote longevity and health, including a diet rich in nutritious foods, an active lifestyle, a strong sense of community and strong social connections, as well as stress management and a positive mindset.

The nutritional secrets of the centenarian populations present in the Blue Zones include a wide variety of plant foods such as fruits, vegetables, legumes and whole grains, with a moderate consumption of animal proteins and healthy fats. These populations tend to eat a diet rich in antioxidants, vitamins and minerals, with particular attention to moderation and balance of meals. Additionally, they often practice intermittent fasting and adopt dietary practices that promote digestive and metabolic health, thus contributing to their longevity and vitality.

BENEFITS OF A BLUE ZONE DIET

"It's no secret that more plants are the way to go and all blue zones emphasize a plant-based diet," switching to a blue zone diet can have the following benefits: Longevity It has been suggested that people in the blue zone live long and healthy lives (up to 90 and 100). Improving mental health Obviously what you eat can affect your physical health, but it also impacts your mood and mental well-being. This means that, as the Blue Zone Diet demonstrates, the more high-quality whole foods, the better.

THE REGIONS OF LONGEVITY

The Blue Zones are five areas of the world where there is an exceptional concentration of centenarians, i.e. people who live beyond 100 years of age. These areas are:

Ogliastra, Sardinia, Italy: Located in the heart of Sardinia, Ogliastra is famous for its Mediterranean diet rich in fruits, vegetables, legumes, whole grains and fish. The residents of the area are also very physically active and enjoy a strong sense of community.

Okinawa, Japan: Okinawa is an archipelago of islands located south of Japan. Okinawans eat a traditional diet of fermented plant foods, fish and seaweed. They also regularly engage in physical activity, such as tai chi and gardening.

Loma Linda, California, United States: Loma Linda is a Californian city inhabited by a large community of Seventh-day Adventists. Seventh-day Adventists are known for their vegetarian diet, abstention from smoking, and emphasis on exercise and rest.

Nicoya Peninsula, Costa Rica: The Nicoya Peninsula is located on the western coast of Costa Rica. The inhabitants of the peninsula have a diet rich in beans, rice and fruit. They are also very physically active and live in a calm and relaxed environment.

Ikaria, Greece: Ikaria is a Greek island located in the Aegean Sea. The inhabitants of Ikaria follow a Mediterranean diet similar to that of Ogliastra. They are also known for their habit of drinking red wine in moderation and living a stress-free life.

Researchers studying the Blue Zones have found that several factors contribute to the longevity of the inhabitants of these areas, including:

Diet: The diet of the populations of the Blue Zones is rich in fruit, vegetables, legumes, whole grains and fish. These foods are rich in nutrients essential for good health and can help protect against chronic disease.

Physical activity: Blue Zone residents are generally very physically active. They do physical activity regularly, both as part of their daily work and for leisure.

Sense of community: Blue Zone residents enjoy a strong sense of community.

Stress Management: Blue Zone residents have developed healthy mechanisms to manage stress. They practice relaxation techniques such as meditation and yoga and spend time in nature.

Adequate sleep: Blue Zone residents sleep an average of 7-8 hours a night. Adequate sleep is important for physical and mental health.

If you are interested in living a longer, healthier life, you may consider adopting some of the principles of the Blue Zones lifestyle. Eat a diet rich in fruits, vegetables, legumes and whole grains. Do physical activity regularly. Cultivate a sense of community in your life. Manage stress in a healthy way. And make sure you get enough sleep. By following these tips, you can increase your chances of living a long, healthy, and happy life.

THE SECRETS OF THE NUTRITION OF CENTENARY POPULATIONS

The Blue Zones are five regions of the world where people live exceptionally long and healthy lives. These places have attracted the attention of researchers studying factors that contribute to longevity. Nutrition plays a fundamental role in the health and longevity of the inhabitants of the Blue Zones. Their diet is characterized by some key elements:

1. Abundance of plant foods:

Fruit, vegetables, legumes and whole grains are the basis of the diet of centenarian populations. These foods are rich in fiber, vitamins, minerals and antioxidants, which are essential for good health and can help protect against chronic disease.

2. Moderate protein consumption:

Protein is important for health, but Blue Zone residents consume it in moderation. Their preferred protein sources include legumes, fish, eggs and dairy products.

3. Healthy Fats:

Blue Zone residents consume healthy fats from sources such as olives, nuts, avocados and fish. These fats can help improve heart health and reduce the risk of chronic disease.

4. Limiting Refined Sugars and Grains:

Blue Zone residents consume limited amounts of refined sugars and grains. These foods can increase the risk of obesity, diabetes and heart disease.

5. Adequate Hydration:

Water is essential for health and Blue Zone residents drink plenty of water throughout the day.

In addition to these key elements, the diet of centenarian populations is often characterized by:

Fresh, Seasonal Food: Blue Zoners eat fresh, seasonal foods that are rich in nutrients.

Home Cooking: Most Blue Zoners cook their meals at home, which allows them to control the ingredients and cooking method.

Slow, Mindful Meals: Blue Zoners enjoy their meals slowly and mindfully, which can help improve digestion and nutrient absorption.

A sense of community: Meals are often an opportunity to gather with family and friends, which can provide a sense of belonging and social support.

By following the dietary principles of centenarian populations, you can improve your health and increase your chances of living a long, healthy life.

Remember that nutrition is only one factor that contributes to longevity. Other important factors include physical activity, stress management, adequate sleep and a positive attitude.

With a little effort and dedication, you can adopt some of the Blue Zones dietary principles into your life and start reaping the benefits to your health and well-being.

THE FUNDAMENTAL PRINCIPLES OF THE BLUE ZONE DIET

The Blue Zone Diet is inspired by the eating habits of people living in the Blue Zones, five areas of the world with the highest concentration of centenarians. These principles are based on a diet rich in plant foods, low in saturated fats and added sugars, and moderate in calories. Here are the fundamental principles of the Blue Zone Diet:

1. Emphasis on plant foods:

Fruits and vegetables: They should form the basis of your diet.

Legumes: Lentils, beans and chickpeas are excellent sources of plant-based protein, fiber and minerals.

Whole grains: Choose whole grains like brown rice, quinoa and oats instead of refined grains.

Nuts and seeds: They are a good source of healthy fats, protein and fiber.

2. Lean Protein:

Consume moderate amounts of lean protein from sources such as fish, poultry, legumes, and low-fat dairy products. Limit red and processed meats.

3. Healthy Fats:

Choose healthy fats such as those from olive oil, avocados, nuts and seeds. Limit saturated and trans fats.

4. Limit added sugars:

Reduce consumption of refined sugar, syrups and artificial sweeteners. Choose fresh fruits and vegetables as a natural source of sweetness.

5. Calorie moderation:

Eat until you are full, but avoid binging. Pay attention to portion sizes to maintain a healthy body weight.

Other important tips: Drink plenty of water: It is important to stay hydrated throughout the day. Cooking at home: Cooking at home allows you to control the ingredients and cooking method. Eat slow, mindful meals: Take time to enjoy your food and savor every bite. Exercise regularly: Physical activity is important for your overall health and can help you live longer. Manage stress: Chronic stress can have a negative impact on your health. Find healthy ways to manage stress, such as meditation or yoga. Get enough sleep: Adequate sleep is important for physical and mental health. By following these basic principles, you can improve your health and increase your chances of living a long, healthy life. Remember that the Blue Zone Diet is not a strict diet, but rather a lifestyle. It's about making healthy food choices and adopting habits that promote longevity and well-being.

THE SCIENTIFIC BASIS OF THE BLUE ZONE DIET

The Blue Zone Diet is based on decades of scientific research demonstrating the benefits of a plant-based, nutrient-rich, calorie-moderate diet for health and longevity.

Here are some of the main scientific evidences that support the Blue Zone Diet:

1. Reduced risk of chronic diseases:

Heart Disease: The Blue Zone Diet is associated with a lower risk of heart disease, the leading cause of death worldwide. This is thanks to the high consumption of fruits, vegetables, legumes and whole grains, which are rich in fiber, vitamins, minerals and antioxidants that can help reduce blood pressure, LDL ("bad") cholesterol and the risk of heart attack.

Stroke: The Blue Zone Diet is also associated with a lower risk of stroke. This is thanks to high consumption of fruits, vegetables and fish, which are rich in nutrients that can help improve blood circulation and reduce the risk of blood clots.

Type 2 diabetes: The Blue Zone Diet can help prevent or manage type 2 diabetes. This is thanks to the high consumption of fiber and low consumption of added sugars, which help regulate blood sugar levels.

Cancer: Some research suggests that the Blue Zone Diet may help reduce the risk of certain types of cancer, such as colon cancer and breast cancer. This is thanks to the high consumption of fruit, vegetables, legumes and whole grains, which are rich in plant compounds with anti-tumor properties.

2. Increased Longevity:

Studies on Blue Zones: Studies conducted in Blue Zones have shown that the inhabitants of these regions have a longer average lifespan than the global average. This has been attributed in part to their diet, which is high in plant foods and low in saturated fats and added sugars. Research on specific foods: Some research suggests that consuming certain foods, such as fruits, vegetables, legumes and nuts, may be associated with a lower risk of death and increased longevity.

3. Improved Mental Health:

Diet and mood: Some research suggests that a healthy diet can improve mood and reduce the risk of depression.

This is thanks to the high consumption of fruit, vegetables and fish, which are rich in nutrients that can positively influence the production of neurotransmitters in the brain. Diet and cognitive function: Some research suggests that a healthy diet can help improve cognitive function and reduce the risk of cognitive decline and dementia. This is thanks to the high consumption of fruit, vegetables, legumes and whole grains, which are rich in nutrients important for brain health.

It is important to highlight that the Blue Zone Diet is just one factor that contributes to health and longevity. Other important factors include physical activity, stress management, adequate sleep and a positive attitude.

BALANCE MACRO NUTRIENTS

The Blue Zone Diet emphasizes a plant-based, nutrient-rich, calorie-moderate diet, rather than specifically counting macronutrients (carbohydrates, proteins, fats). However, balancing macronutrients can still be helpful in feeling full and providing your body with the energy it needs. Here are some considerations on balancing macronutrients within the Blue Zone Diet:

1. Emphasis on complex carbohydrates:

The Blue Zone Diet focuses on fruits, vegetables, legumes and whole grains. These foods are naturally rich in complex carbohydrates, which release energy slowly and help keep blood sugar levels stable.

Aim to consume most of your carbohydrates from whole plant sources instead of refined sources like white bread, white pasta and white rice.

2. Moderate Protein:

The Blue Zone Diet encourages the inclusion of lean protein sources such as fish, poultry, legumes and low-fat dairy products.

The amount of protein you need depends on various factors such as age, gender, activity level and health goals. In general, the average person needs about 0.8 grams of protein per pound of body weight per day.

3. Healthy Fats:

The Blue Zone Diet encourages the inclusion of healthy fats from olive oil, avocado, nuts and seeds. These fats are essential for heart health, brain health and for absorbing some fat-soluble vitamins.

An easy way to balance macronutrients on the Blue Zone Diet is to follow the healthy eating plan: Half your plate: Fill half your plate with fruits and vegetables. Quarter of your plate: Fill a quarter of your plate with whole grains like brown rice, quinoa or oats. Quarter of your plate: Fill the last quarter of your plate with lean protein or healthy fats. This method will naturally help you consume the majority of your carbohydrates from plant sources and include moderate amounts of protein and healthy fats. Also: Eat until you're full, but avoid bingeing. There's no need to rigidly count calories: The Blue Zone Diet focuses on healthy food choices rather than calorie restriction. Consult a nutritionist: If you have concerns or need a personalized plan, consult a registered nutritionist who can help you balance macronutrients based on your individual needs.

IMPLEMENT THE BLUE ZONE LIFESTYLE

Adopting the Blue Zone lifestyle goes beyond just diet. It's about incorporating habits that promote longevity and overall well-being. Here are some steps to implement the Blue Zone lifestyle into your daily life:

1. Power:

Follow the principles of the Blue Zone Diet:

Increase your consumption of fruit, vegetables, legumes and whole grains.

Include lean protein sources such as fish, poultry, legumes and low-fat dairy products.

Choose healthy fats from olive oil, avocado, nuts and seeds.

Limit added sugars, refined grains and red meats.

Plan your weekly meals and prepare meals in advance for greater adherence.

2. Physical activity:

Be active every day:

You don't need to join a gym. Walking, cycling, swimming, dancing or gardening are great activities.

Aim for at least 30 minutes of moderate physical activity most days of the week.

Find an activity that you enjoy and can integrate into your daily routine.

3. Purpose in life:

Having a sense of purpose and meaning in life is crucial.

Find something that you are passionate about and that motivates you to get up every morning.

It can be a job you love, a creative hobby, or volunteering.

Having goals and plans for the future can help you stay motivated and positive.

4. Manage stress:

Find healthy ways to manage stress, such as meditation, yoga, tai chi, or simply spending time in nature. Learn to say no when necessary and delegate tasks when possible.

Deep breathing practices and relaxation techniques can help you manage daily stress.

5. Sense of community:

Cultivating positive, strong relationships is important for health and well-being.

Spend time with family and friends who support you and make you feel good. Get involved in your community.

Feeling part of something bigger than yourself can contribute to a longer, happier life.

6. Adequate sleep: Aim to sleep 7 to 8 hours a night. Create a regular and relaxing sleep routine. Avoid bright screens and stimulating activities before bed.

7. Long-term commitment:

Adopting the Blue Zone lifestyle is a long-term commitment. Don't expect immediate results. Focus on making small, sustainable changes to your daily routine.

Celebrate your successes and don't be discouraged by missteps.

Remember that every small positive change will contribute to your long-term health and longevity.

Also: Implementing the Blue Zone lifestyle isn't about becoming perfect. It's about making positive choices for your health and well-being every day. With a little hard work and dedication, you can live a longer, healthier, happier life.

CONCLUSIONS - THE FUTURE OF THE BLUE ZONE DIET

The Blue Zone Diet is based on solid scientific foundations and offers a practical and realistic approach to a longer, healthier life. Here are some of the reasons why the Blue Zone Diet is here to stay:

It is based on whole, nutritious foods: The Blue Zone Diet emphasizes the consumption of fruits, vegetables, legumes, whole grains and lean proteins, all foods rich in nutrients essential for health. Promotes a Healthy Lifestyle: In addition to diet, the Blue Zone Diet encourages regular physical activity, stress management, adequate sleep, and cultivating positive social relationships, all of which contribute to longevity and overall well-being. It is flexible and adaptable: The Blue Zone Diet is not a rigid diet, but rather a flexible guide that can be adapted to individual needs and preferences.

It's delicious and enjoyable: There are endless delicious and nutritious recipes that fit the principles of the Blue Zone Diet. It's supported by scientific evidence: The Blue Zone Diet is supported by a growing body of scientific research demonstrating its health benefits and longevity.

As research on the Blue Zone Diet advances and more people adopt its principles, its impact on public health will likely increase. The Blue Zone Diet has the potential to reduce the incidence of chronic disease, improve quality of life and increase life expectancy worldwide. In addition to its individual application, the Blue Zone Diet can also be used to inform population-level policies and interventions. Promoting plant-based diets, encouraging physical activity and creating environments that promote socialization and stress management can have a positive impact on the health and well-being of entire communities.

Ultimately, the future of the Blue Zone Diet is bright. With its emphasis on whole foods, a healthy lifestyle, and the pursuit of wellness, the Blue Zone Diet offers a promising path to a longer, healthier, happier life for everyone. In addition to the above, here are some additional points to consider: Ongoing Research: Research on the Blue Zone Diet is constantly evolving and more and more health benefits are being discovered. New technologies: New technologies can be used to make the Blue Zone Diet more accessible and personalized. Education and awareness: It is important to raise awareness of the benefits of the Blue Zone Diet and provide people with the resources needed to adopt it. Together, these factors can help make the Blue Zone Diet a powerful force for improving the health and well-being of people around the world.

FINAL TIPS FOR EMBRACING A HEALTHY AND LONG LASTING LIFESTYLE

Final advice for embracing a healthy and long-lasting lifestyle

Adopting a healthy and long-lasting lifestyle is not an impossible task. It's about making conscious, positive choices every day. Here are some final tips to help you get started:

1. Start with small steps: You don't need to turn your life upside down overnight. Start with small changes that you can sustain over time. For example, you can start adding more fruits and vegetables to your diet, take a daily walk, or dedicate 10 minutes a day to meditation.

2. Find your motivation: What drives you to want to live a healthier and longer life? Having a clear goal can help you stay motivated in the long term.

3. Realize the benefits: Take time to learn about the benefits of a healthy lifestyle. This will help you stay focused on your goals and overcome challenges you may encounter along the way.

4. Don't be discouraged by missteps: Everyone makes mistakes. If you fail, don't give up. Simply start where you left off.

5. Find support: Surround yourself with people who support you on your journey to a healthy lifestyle. This could include family, friends, a support group or a nutritionist.

6. Listen to your body: Pay attention to your body's signals. If you feel tired, stressed or fatigued, take time to rest and recharge.

7. Have fun! A healthy lifestyle doesn't have to be boring. Find ways to have fun while making healthy choices.

Remember, the healthy and long-lived lifestyle is a journey, not a destination. Enjoy the process and celebrate your successes along the way. In addition to the tips above, here are some resources you may find helpful: With a little hard work and dedication, you can live a longer, healthier, happier life.

RECIPES APPETIZERS

WHITE BEAN SALAD WITH TOMATOES AND ONIONS

Preparation time: 10 minutes

Cooking time: N/A

Doses for 4 people:

Ingredients:

Cooked white beans: 200 g

Tomato: 1 medium

Red onion: 1/2

Olive oil: 1 tbsp

Lemon juice: 1 tbsp

Salt to taste

Pepper as needed

Preparation:

Rinse the cooked white beans under running water. Cut the tomato into cubes and the red onion into thin slices. In a large bowl, combine the white beans, tomato, red onion, olive oil, lemon juice, salt and pepper. Mix well to combine the ingredients. Serve the salad immediately or store in the refrigerator for up to 2 days.

TOMATO AND MOZZARELLA SKEWERS

Preparation time: 5 minutes

Cooking time: N/A

Doses for 4 people:

Ingredients:

Tomato: 1 medium

Fresh mozzarella: 1

Fresh basil: 12 leaves

Olive oil: 1 tbsp

Salt to taste

Pepper as needed

Preparation:

Cut the tomato and mozzarella into cubes. Wash the basil leaves. On a skewer, alternate the tomatoes, mozzarella and basil leaves. Drizzle with olive oil, salt and pepper. Serve the skewers immediately.

HUMMUS WITH FRESH VEGETABLES

Preparation time: 15 minutes

Cooking time: N/A

Doses for 4 people:

Ingredients:

Cooked chickpeas: 400 g

Tahini: 1/4 cup

Lemon juice: 1/4 cup

Garlic: 2 cloves

Water: 1/4 cup

Olive oil: 1/4 cup

Salt to taste

Pepper as needed

Fresh vegetables: carrots, celery, peppers (to taste)

Preparation:

Rinse the cooked chickpeas under running water. In a food processor, blend the chickpeas, tahini, lemon juice, garlic, water and olive oil until smooth and creamy. Add salt and pepper to taste. Serve the hummus with fresh vegetables cut into sticks.

BOILED EGGS WITH AVOCADO

Preparation time: 10 minutes

Cooking time: 10 minutes

Doses for 4 people:

Ingredients:

Eggs: 4

Avocado: 2

Salt to taste

Pepper as needed

Preparation:

Cook eggs in boiling water for 10 minutes, or until desired doneness. Shell the eggs and cut them in half. Slice the avocados. Garnish the hard-boiled eggs with avocado, salt and pepper. Serve immediately.

QUINOA SALAD WITH GRILLED VEGETABLES

Preparation time: 20 minutes

Cooking time: 15 minutes for quinoa,

15-20 minutes for grilled vegetables

Doses for 4 people:

Ingredients:

Quinoa: 1 cup

Water or vegetable broth: 2 cups

Courgette: 1 medium

Eggplant: 1 medium

Red pepper: 1

Red onion: 1

Olive oil: 3 tablespoons

Salt to taste

Pepper as needed

Preparation:

Rinse the quinoa under running water. In a medium saucepan, cook the quinoa in the water or vegetable broth over low heat for 15 minutes, or until the liquid is absorbed. In the meantime, cut the courgettes, aubergines, peppers and red onion into small pieces. Heat the olive oil in a grill pan over medium-high heat. Grill vegetables for 15 to 20 minutes, turning occasionally, until tender and lightly charred. Drain the cooked quinoa and let it cool slightly. In a large bowl, combine the cooled quinoa, grilled vegetables, salt and pepper. Mix well to combine the ingredients. Serve the salad immediately.

CHICKPEA SALAD WITH FENNEL AND ORANGE

Preparation time: 15 minutes

Cooking time: N/A

Doses for 4 people:

Ingredients:

Cooked chickpeas: 200 g

Fennel: 1 medium

Orange: 1

Olive oil: 1/4 cup

Lemon juice: 2 tablespoons

Balsamic vinegar: 1 tbsp

Salt to taste

Pepper as needed

Preparation:

Rinse the cooked chickpeas under running water. Cut the fennel into thin slices and the orange into segments. In a large bowl, combine the chickpeas, fennel, orange, olive oil, lemon juice, balsamic vinegar, salt and pepper. Mix well to combine the ingredients. Serve the salad immediately or store in the refrigerator for up to 2 days.

MELON WITH FETA AND MINT

Preparation time: 10 minutes

Cooking time: N/A

Doses for 4 people:

Ingredients:

Melon: 1/2

Feta: 200 g

Fresh mint: 1/4 cup

Olive oil: 1 tbsp

Salt to taste

Pepper as needed

Preparation:

Cut the melon into slices, remove the seeds and peel. Cut the feta into cubes. Finely chop the mint leaves. In a bowl, combine the sliced melon, diced feta, chopped mint, olive oil, salt and pepper. Stir gently to combine the ingredients. Serve the melon salad with feta and mint immediately or place in the refrigerator for up to 2 days.

HAM AND RICOTTA ROLLS

Preparation time: 15 minutes

Cooking time: N/A

Doses for 4 people:

Ingredients:

Raw ham: 8 slices

Ricotta: 250 g

Chopped fresh herbs:

1/4 cup (basil,

parsley, chives)

Salt to taste

Pepper as needed

Preparation:

In a bowl, mix the ricotta with the chopped fresh herbs, salt and pepper. Spread the slices of raw ham on a work surface. Spread a spoonful of the ricotta mixture on each slice of ham. Roll the ham slices to form rolls. Cut the rolls in half diagonally. Serve the ham and ricotta rolls immediately or place them in the refrigerator for up to 2 days.

GRILLED VEGETABLES WITH TZATZIKI SAUCE

Preparation time: 20 minutes

Cooking time: 15 minutes

for the grilled vegetables,

10 minutes for the tzatziki sauce

Doses for 4 people:

Ingredients:

Zucchini: 2 medium

Eggplant: 1 medium

Red pepper: 1

Red onion: 1

Olive oil: 3 tablespoons

Salt to taste

Pepper as needed

Ingredients for the tzatziki sauce:

Greek yogurt: 200 g

Cucumber: 1 medium

Garlic: 1 clove

Fresh dill: 1/4 cup

Lemon juice: 1 tbsp

Salt to taste

Pepper as needed

Preparation:

For the grilled vegetables: Cut the courgettes, aubergines, peppers and red onion into small pieces. Heat the olive oil in a grill pan over medium-high heat. Grill the vegetables for 15 minutes, turning occasionally, until tender and slightly charred.

Drain the grilled vegetables and let them cool slightly. For the tzatziki sauce: In a bowl, combine the Greek yogurt, grated cucumber, minced garlic, chopped fresh dill, lemon juice, salt and pepper. Mix well to combine the ingredients. Cover the tzatziki sauce and refrigerate for at least 30 minutes before serving. To compose the dish: Arrange the grilled vegetables on a serving plate. Pour the tzatziki sauce over the grilled vegetables. Serve immediately.

AVOCADO AND SMOKED SALMON CANAPÉS

Preparation time: 10 minutes

Cooking time: N/A

Doses for 4 people:

Ingredients:

Wholemeal bread: 8 slices

Avocado: 2 ripe

Smoked salmon: 200 g

Lemon juice: 1/4 cup

Salt to taste

Pepper as needed

Preparation:

Toast the slices of wholemeal bread. Mash the avocados in a bowl and drizzle with lemon juice to prevent them from blackening. Spread the toasted avocado on each slice of bread. Arrange the smoked salmon on the avocado tartlets. Season with salt and pepper to taste. Serve the avocado and smoked salmon canapés immediately.

GUACAMOLE

Difficulty: Very easy

Preparation: 20 min

Doses for: 6 people

Low cost

ingredients

Avocado (2) 500 g

White onions (half) 35 g

Lime juice 35 g

Coriander to taste

Copper tomatoes 1

Salt up to 1 pinch

Preparation

To prepare the guacamole, first peel and finely chop the onion 1, then also chop the coriander 2. Divide the avocado in half and remove the stone 3. Remove the pulp with the help of a spoon and pour it inside of a mortar 4. Add the lime juice 5 and start crushing until you obtain a cream 6. Also add the chopped onion 7 and the coriander 8 and crush again to mix everything together, then add the salt 9. If you like spicy foods, at this point you can add fresh chilli pepper or a few drops of Tabasco. Finally, cut the tomato into cubes 10 and add it to the sauce 11. Your guacamole sauce is ready to be served.

TUNA AND POTATO MEATBALLS

Difficulty: Easy

Preparation: 25 min

Cooking: 45 min

Doses for: 15 pieces

ingredients

Drained natural tuna 110 g

Potatoes 650 g

Thyme to taste

Sage to taste

Salt to taste

Black pepper to taste

Lemon zest 1

For breading and frying

Eggs 2

Breadcrumbs 150 g

Seed oil to taste

Preparation

To prepare the tuna and potato meatballs, first boil the potatoes in cold water 1 for about 40 minutes 2. This time varies according to the size of the potatoes. To check that they are cooked, try pricking them with a fork, if the tines they will go in easily meaning they are cooked. At this point, drain and peel them; then mash them in a bowl, using the appropriate tool 3. Let them cool and in the meantime prepare the chopped thyme and sage 4. As soon as the potatoes are no longer hot, add the tuna, the aromatic chopped 5, and season with salt 6. Add the pepper 7 and the grated zest of a lemon 8 and mix everything together with a fork 9 until you obtain a uniform mixture. At this point prepare meatballs weighing approximately 25 g 10, then dip first in the beaten egg 11 and then in the breadcrumbs 12. In the meantime, while preparing the meatballs, pour the oil into a pan and heat it until it reaches temperature of 170°. As soon as this is hot enough, dive in a few pieces at a time 14. Fry the tuna and potato meatballs for about 3 minutes, then drain them with a slotted spoon and transfer to a sheet of frying paper 14. Finish frying and serve your meatballs of tuna and boiling potatoes 15.

SPRING ROLLS

Difficulty: Easy

Preparation: 30 min

Cooking: 20 min

Doses for: 8 pieces

Average cost

ingredients

Sheets in roll (21.5 x 21.5 cm) 8 sheets

Cabbage) 300 g Carrots 60 g, White onions 50 g

Rice wine 30 g, peanut oil to taste

Salt to taste

White (or black) pepper to taste

Egg whites to taste

Peanut seed oil

Preparation

To prepare the spring rolls, first defrost the ready-made sheets of pastry and cover them with a slightly damp cloth to prevent them from drying out. Peel and cut the cabbage 1, the onions 2 and the carrots 3 into thin strips. Heat the wok over a high heat, then pour in the vegetable oil and the onions 4. Fry for a couple of minutes, then add the carrots and the cabbage 5. Season with salt and pepper 6. Also add the rice wine 7 and brown the vegetables for 4-5 minutes: they must be cooked but still crunchy 8. Transfer the vegetables into a colander to eliminate any excess liquids, then spread them a little with chopsticks to better preserve color and consistency 10.

Fold the lower corner upwards and roll without pressing until the filling is covered 11, then fold the corners on the sides towards the center 12. Finally, roll the roll from the bottom upwards 13 and seal the pastry by slightly moistening the edges with a little egg white 14, you can use your fingers or a brush. Don't press too hard or the dough may break. Proceed in this way to form all the rolls 15. Now heat the wok again, then pour plenty of seed oil 16 to bring it to a temperature of 180°. When the oil is hot, lower the heat slightly and fry a few rolls at a time 17, turning them on both sides 18. When they are golden brown on both sides, drain the rolls 19 and place them on kitchen paper to absorb the excess oil 20. Serve your spring rolls while still hot accompanied by spicy or sweet and sour sauce!

VITELLO TONNATO

Difficulty: Easy

Preparation: 30 min

Cooking: 55 min

Doses for: 4 people

Cost: High

ingredients

Veal (round or silverside) 800 g

Celery 1 rib

Carrots 1

Golden onions 1

Garlic 1 clove

White wine 250 g

Water 1.5l

Extra virgin olive oil 3 tablespoons

Black peppercorns to taste

Salt to taste

For the sauce, 2 eggs

Tuna in oil, drained 100 g

Anchovies in oil 3 fillets

Salted capers 5 g

Caper fruits to decorate to taste

Meat broth 150 g

Preparation

To prepare the veal with tuna sauce, start by cleaning the vegetables that will be used to cook the meat. Wash them, then peel the carrot and clean it, cut it into small pieces. Then remove the ends of the celery and cut it into small pieces 1. Peel the onion and divide it into 2 parts, clean the garlic and serve it whole. Move on to cleaning the meat, eliminating any cartilage and fat strands. 2. Place the piece of silverside 3 in a large pot. Add the chopped vegetables and 4 garlic and black peppercorns. Pour the white wine 7 and then the water 8 which must cover everything. Season with salt and then add the oil. 9. Turn on the stove and wait for it to boil. Gradually remove the foam that comes to the surface 10. Then close the lid and lower the heat slightly, leaving to cook for around 40-45 minutes: remembering that for every 500 g of meat it takes around 30 minutes of cooking. The important thing is that the heart of the meat does not exceed 65°, to be measured with a kitchen thermometer. Once the piece of meat is cooked, drain it 11 and let it cool completely 12. Then filter the broth 13. You will need about 150 g of broth. In the meantime, prepare the hard-boiled eggs. In a saucepan with plenty of cold water,

Turn on the stove and count 9 minutes from the moment of boiling. Once they have hardened, drain them and rinse under cold water. Once cooled, peel them and cut them into 4 parts 15. In a bowl, pour the egg segments, the drained tuna 16, the anchovies in oil 17, and the desalted capers, finally add the broth little by little 19. Use the blender to submerge and add more broth if necessary. Blend 20 until you obtain a smooth cream 21. At this point the meat must be completely cold. Slice thinly with a smooth-bladed knife 22. Arrange the slices on a serving plate and pour the cream obtained in the center 24. Finally decorate with the caper fruits, some whole and others cut in half and your vitello with tuna sauce is ready.

SCALLOPS GRATINATE

Difficulty: Very easy

Preparation: 15 min

Cooking: 15 min

Doses for: 4 people

Average cost

ingredients

Scallops 8

Grated bread 100 g

Black pepper to taste

Salt to taste

Extra virgin olive oil 40 g

Lemon zest 1, Parsley to taste

Thyme to taste

Marjoram to taste

Preparation

To gratinate the scallops, start with the breadcrumbs: take the breadcrumbs and remove the crust (you can make crunchy croutons with the crust you have removed); cut the breadcrumbs into cubes 1. Transfer it to a mixer, add the oil 2, salt and pepper to taste 3, add the aromatic herbs, parsley, marjoram and thyme (4-5), and finally grate the lemon zest 6. Blend and you will obtain manure 7; with these doses your panure will be moist at the right point, so that the result is tasty and does not remain too dry. Take the scallops and place them on a baking tray, with the shell facing the base so as to fill the scallops with the panure obtained 8. Once distributed, cook them in a preheated ventilated oven at 190° for about 15 minutes or just as an inviting crust 9. Your scallops au gratin are ready to be served!

SPINACH AND RICOTTA MEATBALLS

Difficulty: Very easy

Preparation: 25 min

Cooking: 25 min

Doses for: 24 pieces

Low cost

ingredients

Already cleaned spinach 250 g

Cow's milk ricotta 250 g

Parmesan to grate 50 g

Breadcrumbs 40 g

Extra virgin olive oil 20 g

Garlic 1 clove

Salt to taste

Black pepper to taste, for breading

1 eggs, breadcrumbs to taste

Salt to taste, Black pepper to taste

Preparation

To prepare the spinach and ricotta meatballs, start by heating the oil together with a whole clove of garlic 1, immerse the previously washed spinach and let it sizzle over a high heat, cooking for 5-6 minutes and stirring often 2 until they soften completely 3 Remove the garlic 4 and then put the spinach to drain in a colander, crushing them slightly with a spatula so as to lose the excess water and leave to cool like this 5; once cold, chop coarsely with a knife 6. At this point, pour the ricotta into a bowl (if there is a lot of water, drain it first) and mix with the spoon 7, then add the spinach and the grated cheese 8, season with salt and pepper, and knead 9. Then, to give the meatballs more consistency, add the breadcrumbs 10 and continue kneading 11. As soon as the dough is ready you can start forming the meatballs. Then take a little dough, about 20 grams, and shape it with your hands 12; you will thus obtain approximately 24-26 meatballs 13. Gradually then pass them delicately into a small bowl in which you have beaten the egg together with salt and pepper 14, and then into another small bowl in which there will be the breadcrumbs 15. Continue in this way until you finish them all and arrange them one by one on a baking tray lined with baking paper (16-17). Cook the spinach and ricotta meatballs in a preheated oven, in static mode, at 200° for about 20 minutes. Serve them piping hot!

CRISPY POTATO PANCAKES

Difficulty: Easy

Preparation: 20 min

Cooking: 20 min

Doses for: 20 pieces

Cost: Very low

ingredients

Potatoes (large) 4

00 flour 2 tbsp

Rosemary 2 sprigs

Salt to taste

Black pepper to taste

Olive oil to taste

Preparation

Wash and peel the potatoes, then cut them into strips 1 (if you have one you can use a special grater) and place them in a bowl. Add a couple of tablespoons of flour 2 to the coarsely chopped rosemary needles 3, and mix to combine the ingredients. Add the pepper 4 and the salt. Pour a couple of fingers of oil into a pan and let it heat up (180°), then take spoonfuls of the mixture and place them in the hot oil, flattening the pancake with the tines of a fork. Brown the pancake on both sides 6 and then drain the excess oil on kitchen paper. Serve the crispy potato pancakes while still hot.

SWEET AND SOUR ONIONS

Difficulty: Very easy

Preparation: 5 min

Cooking: 40 min

Doses for: 4 people, Low cost

ingredients

Borettane onions 600 g

Apple cider vinegar 40 g

Brown sugar 40 g, Butter 30 g

Water 15 g, Thyme 1 sprig

Salt to taste

Black pepper to taste

Preparation

To prepare the sweet and sour onions, pour 1 brown sugar and 2 water into a saucepan. Melt the sugar over low heat, mix with a wooden spoon, then add the butter 3. When the butter has also melted, add the onions that you have previously washed 4, salted 5 and peppered. Cook for a couple of minutes over medium heat, stirring often to cover them evenly with the glaze 6. Now add the vinegar 7. Allow the strong smell of the vinegar to evaporate without allowing the liquid to dry 8, then add the thyme 9 Cover with a lid and cook over medium-low heat for 30 minutes, stirring occasionally 10; if they dry out or become too colored you can wet them with a little water. After this time, check that the onions are tender 11; if you want a more buttery consistency you can continue cooking for another 10 minutes. To further thicken the icing you can add a knob of cold butter at the end of cooking. Your sweet and sour onions are ready!

FISH BALLS

Difficulty: Easy

Preparation: 30 min

Cooking: 4 min

Doses for: 20 pieces

Average cost

ingredients

Cod fillet 700 g,

Grated bread 100 g

Parsley 1 sprig, Thyme to taste

Eggs (medium) 2, Garlic 1 clove

Salt to taste

Black pepper to taste

Parmesan to grate 80 g

00 flour to taste, peanut oil to taste

Preparation

To prepare the fish balls, start by placing the breadcrumbs in a blender 1, blending finely 2, and placing it in a bowl. Remove the bones from the cod fillets with the help of tweezers and chop them in the mixer for a few seconds 3. Mix the chopped cod with the bread in a bowl 4. Wash and chop the parsley 5, then add it to the bowl 6 together with the thyme. Season with the crushed garlic 7 and the grated cheese 8. Then add the two eggs 9. Season with salt 10 and pepper. Stir well to mix everything 11 and with yours

With your hands, form balls the size of a walnut with about 30 g of dough 12. Gradually arrange the meatballs on a tray, and you will get about 20-25 13. Then dip in the flour 14-15. Fry the meatballs 2/3 times in very hot seed oil, at around 170°, for around 3 minutes. When the meatballs are golden, drain them from the oil with the help of a slotted spoon 16 and place them on absorbent paper 17 to dry the excess oil. Enjoy fish balls hot or warm!

AUBERGINES ROLLS

Difficulty: Very easy

Preparation: 15 min

Cooking: 30 min

Doses for: 12 pieces

Cost: Very low

ingredients

Aubergines 650 g

Cooked Ham 225 g

Tomato puree 400 g

Extra virgin olive oil to taste

Salt to taste

Black pepper to taste

Provola 225 g

Garlic 1 clove

Basil to taste

Preparation

To prepare the aubergine rolls, first wash and dry the aubergines, then remove the stems and cut them lengthwise with a mandolin to obtain 15 slices about 1 cm thick. 1. Arrange the aubergine slices on a baking tray lined with baking paper, oil, 2 salt and pepper. Now cook 3 in a preheated fan oven at 210 degrees for 10 minutes. In the meantime, prepare the tomato sauce. Pour a drizzle of oil and a clove of garlic into a saucepan.

Pour the tomato puree, add salt and flavor with basil, bring to the boil, lower the temperature and cook for about 20 minutes. Once the aubergines are cooked, start stuffing them with the cheese 7 and the cooked ham 8. Roll up to obtain the rolls 9. Keep the rolls aside 10. Pour 2-3 tablespoons of tomato puree into a baking tray 11, and arrange the eggplant rolls 12 next to each other. Cover the aubergines with the rest of the sauce 13. Cook for 20 minutes in a preheated oven in static mode at 200°. Once cooked, serve the aubergine rolls hot and stringy!

RECIPES
FIRST DISHES

ORECCHIETTE, TURNIP TOPS AND GINGER

Time 25 min

ingredients

4 people

500 g of fresh orecchiette

320 g of cleaned turnip greens

garlic

fresh ginger

extra virgin olive oil

salt

Pepper

Preparation

For the orecchiette, turnip tops and ginger recipe, blanch the turnip tops in boiling salted water for 30 seconds and drain them with a slotted spoon. Boil the orecchiette in the same water as the turnip tops. Chop the tops and brown them in a pan with 3 tablespoons of oil, 1 clove of garlic and 1 teaspoon of grated ginger. When they start to sizzle, wet them with 1 ladle of the pasta cooking water. Drain the orecchiette and season them directly in the pan with the tops, complete with freshly ground pepper.

SPAGHETTI WITH CLAMS WITH PUMPKIN SAUCE

Time 1h 10 min + 2h rest

ingredients

Portions for 4 people

1.4 kg clams

300 grams of spaghetti

200 g of diced pumpkin pulp

50 g of onion

4 mustard leaves

parsley

garlic salt

extra virgin olive oil

Preparation

For the spaghetti with clams recipe with pumpkin sauce and mandarin mustard, soak the clams in 2 liters of water with 40 g of salt for a couple of hours. Rinse well, beating, to remove all the sand. Heat 100 g of oil in a pan with 3 g of chopped garlic; when the garlic starts to come to the surface, add the clams, cover with a lid and let them open over a low heat. Drain the clams from the cooking water, filter it and keep it aside. Shell the clams and season them with 2 g of chopped parsley. Chop the onion and simmer it with 50 g of oil for 3-4 minutes;

Add the pumpkin, cover with water and cook for 20-25 minutes, until soft. Blend with 50 g of water and season with salt. Cook the spaghetti in plenty of salted water for about 6 minutes (for 2/3 of the cooking time indicated on the package); finish cooking the spaghetti in the pan in about 3 minutes, wetting them like a risotto with the filtered clam water, then add the shelled clams. Distribute the pumpkin sauce on the plates; place the spaghetti with clams on top, complete with the strips of mustard leaves and serve.

HALF SLEEVES WITH RED BEETS

Time 35 min

ingredients

Servings for 6 people

300 g of red and yellow beets

100 g of milk, salt

150 grams of cream

60 g of sliced cooked ham

600 g of half sleeved pasta

Preparation

For the red beetroot half sleeves recipe, bring the milk and cream to the boil in a saucepan and, in another pan, plenty of salted water for the pasta. Wash the beets and separate the leaves from the stems;

Blanch the leaves in the boiling pasta water for 2 minutes, then transfer to the cream and milk mixture, lowering the heat and continuing cooking for 5 minutes. Mix, turn off the heat and blend everything with an immersion blender, obtaining a creamy sauce. Heat a non-stick pan and distribute the coppa slices without overlapping them; roast for a couple of minutes, until crisp, then remove from the pan. Cook the pasta according to the times indicated on the package, together with the colored stems of the chard cut into small pieces; drain, transfer everything to the pan where you browned the coppa, and stir in the chard sauce. Distribute the half sleeves on the plates, complete with the ham and serve.

SPAGHETTI WITH COD SAUCE

Time 1h 10min

ingredients

Portions for 4 people

400 g of peeled tomatoes

350 grams of spaghetti

350 g of cod, soaked and desalted

4 bran peppers

3 shallots

1 egg

small salted capers

re-milled durum wheat semolina

extra virgin olive oil

white wine, salt

Preparation

For the spaghetti with cod sauce recipe, finely slice the shallot and simmer it gently in a pan with a drizzle of oil; then blend with 1/2 glass of wine, then add the roughly chopped tomatoes and cook the sauce over low heat for 30 minutes. Cut the cabbage into 4-5 cm slices. Dip in the beaten egg, then in the durum wheat semolina, and fry in plenty of oil. Add the cod and capers to the sauce and cook for another 30 minutes. Boil the spaghetti in plenty of salted water. Drain them al dente, using the appropriate ladle, directly into the saucepan and finish cooking, adding a drop of the cooking water if necessary. Fry the brain peppers for 30 seconds in plenty of boiling oil. Drain them, crumble them over the pasta and serve.

CLASSIC TOMATO GNOCCHI

Time 1h 20min

ingredients

Portions for 4 people

1 kg of white pulp potatoes,

250 g of flour

Nutmeg

salt

fresh tomato

basil

Preparation

For the classic tomato gnocchi recipe, wash the potatoes with their peel and cook them the oven at 180°C for 30-35 minutes, covered with aluminum foil. Check the cooking by inserting the tip of the knife; if necessary cook them for another 10-15 minutes. Take them out and let them cool. Form a mound with the flour on the pastry board. Pass the potatoes through a potato masher directly on the flour, add a pinch of salt and a generous grating of nutmeg. Mix quickly to avoid activating the gluten (which would make the gnocchi hard after cooking), obtaining a soft mixture. Form loaves of 2 cm in diameter and divide them into 2-3 cm blocks. Rigatelli by rolling them on the tines of the fork or on the wooden riganocchi. Cook in abundant boiling salted water and drain them for 1 minute after they come to the surface. Season them as you prefer, for example with tomato sauce and basil.

VOGHERESE RISOTTO

Time 45 min

ingredients

Portions for 4 people

1 liter meat broth

320 g of Carnaroli rice

80 grams of butter

80 g grated parmesan

2 Voghera peppers

1 shallot

White wine

salt and pepper

Preparation

For the Vogherese risotto recipe, peel the shallot, chop it and brown it in a saucepan with a knob of butter. Clean the peppers, remove the seeds and white filaments, cut them into lozenges and add them to the pan. Season them for 2 minutes, add a ladle of broth and cook until they have softened and the liquid has evaporated. Take 1 tablespoon of peppers from the pan and set aside to decorate the dish at the end. Toast the rice in the pan with the shallots and peppers, add a splash of white wine and cook the rice, adding the broth little by little. Turn off the heat, season with salt and pepper, then stir in the remaining butter and grated parmesan. Let the risotto rest covered for 5 minutes, then serve it with the reserved peppers and freshly ground pepper.

PASTA WITH ANCHOVIES

Time 50 min

ingredients

4 people

500 g of cherry tomatoes

500 g of very fresh anchovies

300 g of short pasta

2 shallots

fennel

re-milled durum wheat semolina

extra virgin olive oil

Peanut oil

salt

Preparation

For the pasta with anchovies, peel the shallots and cut them in half lengthwise. Slice, always lengthwise, placing the knife blade obliquely to obtain fillets that better retain their structure during cooking. Let them dry gently in a large pan with a thin layer of oil, salt and a few fennel stalks; then add the cherry tomatoes cut in half. Let them soften for 2-3 minutes. Clean the anchovies by opening them like a book, rinse and dry them; Coat them in the re-milled semolina and fry them in peanut oil at 175°C, drain them on kitchen paper as soon as they are golden and crunchy. Boil the pasta, drain it al dente and sauté it over high heat in the pan with the cherry tomatoes. Serve it with fried anchovies and sprigs of fresh fennel.

SPELLED TAGLIOLINI WITH PEPPER SAUCE

Duration 1h 15min

ingredients

4 people

For the tagliolini

150 g of 00 flour

150 g of spelled flour, 3 eggs

1 kg Peppers of various colors

fresh chili pepper, basil, salt

extra virgin olive oil

Preparation

Mix the flours and add them to the eggs, working the mixture until you obtain a homogeneous and smooth mixture. Wrap it in cling film and let it rest for 30 minutes.

Roll out the dough, working little at a time, into thin sheets, with the pasta machine, then cut them into thin slices. Place them on a floured tray. Grease the peppers with a drizzle of oil, place them on a baking tray and bake at 230°C for about 30 minutes, until they are golden. Remove from the oven and let them rest closed in a bag for 10 minutes. Peel them and remove the seeds, making fillets. Cook them for 10 minutes in a saucepan with 1 ladle of water and 1 chopped fresh chilli pepper. Turn off the heat, blend everything and, if you want, pass the cream through a sieve. Cook the cream in a saucepan for 3-5 minutes to thicken; salt it at the end. Boil the tagliolini in boiling salted water for about 3 minutes and drain them into the pan with the sauce. Sauté them briefly and serve, completing with fresh basil leaves.

BUCATINI WITH ZUCCHINI, MINT PESTO AND AVOCADO

Time 35 min

ingredients

Portions for 4 people

360 g bucatini

50 grams of mint

20 g grated parmesan

10 g of pine nuts, 2 courgettes

1 ripe avocado, lemon, ice

extra virgin olive oil

salt, peppercorns

Preparation

For the recipe for courgette bucatini with mint and avocado pesto, boil the bucatini until al dente in salted water.

Drain them and pour them into water and ice to stop the cooking, then drain them very well, eliminating all the water. Cut the courgettes into very thin ribbons, then into spaghetti: use only the green part and keep the rest for the sauce. Dip the courgette fillets in boiling salted water and drain immediately. Blanch the remaining courgettes in boiling salted water, then drain them. Weigh approximately 100g. Clean the mint, keeping only the leaves and blend with the courgettes, grated parmesan, 70-80 g of oil, pine nuts and salt, obtaining a thick pesto. Clean the avocado and blend it with the juice of 1/2 lemon, 1 tablespoon of oil, salt and pepper, obtaining a smooth sauce. Season the pasta with the mint pesto, then mix with the courgette fillets. Serve it with avocado cream and coarsely ground pepper.

LINGUINE WITH GAZPACHO OF BEET, CITRUS FRUITS AND RED PRAWNS

Time 35 min

ingredients

Portions for 4 people

360 g of linguine

250 g 1 boiled beetroot

12 red prawns, 2 lemons

2 pink grapefruits

1 orange, ice

extra virgin olive oil

salt and pepper

Preparation

For the beetroot linguine recipe,

citrus fruits and red prawn gazpacho, boil the linguine al dente in salted water. Drain them and pour them in water and ice to stop the cooking, then drain them very well, eliminating all the water. Blend the beetroot with the juice of 1 lemon, 1 orange, 1 grapefruit and a pinch of salt, for about 5 minutes, until a very smooth mixture is obtained. Shell the prawns and remove the black casing. Season them with a drizzle of oil, salt, pepper and the juice of 1 lemon and leave them to marinate for 2 hours. Season the pasta with the citrus beetroot smoothie, and add all the prawns except the 4, which you will keep for decoration. Serve the pasta with pieces of grapefruit pulp and complete with the remaining prawns. If you like, you can add a little dried and finely crumbled mint.

SPAGHETTI WITH TOMATO BASIL AND ALMOND WATER

Time 40 min

ingredients

Portions for 4 people

360 grams of spaghetti

40 cherry tomatoes

40 fresh almonds

(or shelled without skin)

4 copper tomatoes

ice, basil

extra virgin olive oil

salt and pepper

Preparation

For the spaghetti with tomato, basil and almond water recipe, blanch the tomatoes in boiling water for 30 seconds. Remove the skin, season them with oil, salt, pepper and basil and leave them to marinate in the refrigerator for 12 hours. Boil the spaghetti al dente in salted water. Drain them and pour them into water and ice to stop the cooking, then drain them very well, eliminating all the water. Blend the copper tomatoes and pass the blend through a sieve: lightly crush the pulp, so as to obtain a red tomato water (not completely transparent). Season the spaghetti with this water, complete them with the marinated cherry tomatoes, cut into quarters, and the almonds cut in half. Garnish with basil to taste.

MALLOREDDUS WITH POTATOES, TOMATO AND MINT SAUCE

Time 50 min

ingredients

Portions for 4 people

400 g of potatoes

200 g of dried malloreddus

100 g of sheep's ricotta

100 g of yellow tomato puree

15 g of mint leaves

1 copper tomato

extra virgin olive oil

salt and pepper

Preparation

For the malloreddus recipe with potatoes, tomato and mint sauce, peel the potatoes and cut them into cubes. Heat a drizzle of oil with a pinch of salt in a saucepan and brown the potatoes for 1 minute. Pour in 1 glass of water, bring to the boil and cook for 5-6 minutes. Add the yellow tomato puree and the malloreddus. Cover with water and simmer, with the lid slightly aside, for the cooking time of the pasta. Turn off and season with freshly ground pepper. Work the ricotta with a whisk, making it creamy by adding 1 tablespoon of oil, salt and pepper. Cut the tomato into cubes, removing the part with the seeds. Blanch the mint in boiling salted water, then cool it in water and ice. Drain it and blend it with 100 g of oil. Whitening will keep it bright green. Serve the malloreddus with the ricotta, the diced tomatoes and the mint sauce.

ASPIC SPAGHETTI WITH BLOODY MARYALLE MUSSELS

Time 50 min + 2h rest

ingredients

Portions for 4 people

1 kg of mussels

500 g of peeled tomatoes

360 grams of spaghetti

8 g edible gelatine sheets

lemon, ice, chili pepper, tabasco

extra virgin olive oil

salt and pepper

Preparation

For the recipe for aspic spaghetti with bloody mary with mussels, boil the spaghetti al dente in salted water. Drain and pour them put them in water and ice to stop the cooking, then drain them very well, eliminating all the water. Clean the mussels, then let them open in a saucepan with a drizzle of oil. Shell and filter the cooking water, pepper lightly. Blend the peeled tomatoes and pass them through a sieve to remove impurities and seeds. Soak the gelatin in cold water. Then take 2-3 tablespoons of tomato puree, heat it and dissolve the gelatine, then add the mixture to the rest of the tomato. Also add the filtered water from the mussels and the juice of 1 lemon, the chilli pepper and a splash of Tabasco, obtaining the Bloody Mary. Season the pasta with this Bloody Mary, adding half the mussels. Arrange in 4 molds and let them cool in the refrigerator for 2 hours. Unmold the jellies and serve, completing with the remaining mussels, grated lemon zest,

PENNETTE SALMON AND VODKA

Time 1h

ingredients

4 people

400 g of yellow cherry tomatoes

320 g of penne pasta

200 g of smoked salmon

100g of fresh cream

100g of Greek yogurt

vodka, lime

chives

extra virgin olive oil

salt and pepper

Preparation

For the salmon and vodka penne recipe, coarsely chop the smoked salmon and marinate it for 30 minutes with 4 tablespoons of vodka, 2 tablespoons of lime juice, 2 tablespoons of Greek yogurt and a dozen finely chopped chives. Form small meatballs with the salmon mixture. Cook the penne in boiling salted water, drain 1-2 minutes before the times indicated on the package; season them with a drizzle of oil, spread them on a tray and let them cool. Wash the cherry tomatoes, cut them in half and cook 300 g in a pan with 3 tablespoons of oil and a pinch of salt for 3 minutes.

Blend and sieve them, obtaining a sauce. Cut the remaining cherry tomatoes into small pieces and marinate them with 1 tablespoon of vodka and a pinch of salt for 30 minutes. Whip the cream with a pinch of salt and ground pepper; mix delicately first with the Greek yogurt, mixing from bottom to top, then with half of the yellow cherry tomato sauce, obtaining a cream. Season the pasta with the cream and complete it with the salmon meatballs, the remaining tomato sauce and the marinated cherry tomatoes; season with freshly ground pepper and a few threads of chopped chives and serve.

PACCHERI GRATINATED STUFFED WITH MACKEREL

Time 1h

ingredients

4 people

200 g paccheri

200 g of cleaned mackerel fillets

50 g 2 slices of bread

20 g of red chili pepper

3 copper tomatoes

1 white onion

Parmesan

Oregano, parsley

dry white wine, extra virgin olive oil

salt and pepper

Preparation

For the recipe for paccheri gratin filled with mackerel, cook the paccheri in plenty of salted water: to avoid breaking them, do not boil the water violently and mix gently. Drain them, season them with oil and let them cool. Wash the tomatoes; cut two into 5 mm thick slices and a half into small pieces. Finely blend the bread with 1 teaspoon of oregano and 1 tablespoon of parmesan. Then drizzle with 1 tablespoon of oil. Chop the onion and sauté it in a pan with 2 tablespoons of oil for a couple of minutes; savory. Chop the mackerel fillets. Coarsely chop the pepper with a handful of parsley and add it to the onion; after 1 minute add the wine and 2-3 tablespoons of water;

Cook over medium heat for 3-4 minutes, until the liquid has evaporated. Finally, add the mackerel and cook over medium-low heat for about 5 minutes, until it starts to break down; salt and pepper. Spread onto a cutting board to cool; then chop to obtain the paccheri filling. Season it with a drizzle of oil and knead half the bread. Stuff each pacchero with a couple of teaspoons of filling. Arrange the tomato slices in a baking dish, slightly overlapping, and season them with a drizzle of oil, a pinch of salt and freshly ground pepper. Distribute the leftover filling, the stuffed paccheri and the chopped half tomato over the top. Season with a drizzle of oil and the remaining bread; cook in grill mode for about 4 minutes, until the paccheri are golden.

SEA CARBONARA

Time 1h 15min

ingredients

4 servings

For pasta

250 g of 00 flour

200 g of whole eggs, salt

For the sauce

500 g of cleaned mussels

500 g purged clams

150 g of cleaned squid

100 g of dry white wine

100g of fresh cream

60 g grated parmesan

2 small cloves of garlic

1 whole egg

1 pc yolk

chopped parsley

extra virgin olive oil

Preparation

Mix the flour with the eggs, a pinch of salt and 50-60 g of water, adding it little at a time. Form a loaf, wrap it in baking paper and place it in the fridge to rest for about 30 minutes. Roll out the dough to a thickness of 2 mm and cut out the tagliolini. Place the mussels and clams in a large pan with a sprinkle with oil and the garlic cloves with their peel, brown over high heat for 1 minute, pour in the wine, add 1 tablespoon of parsley and cover; when the shells are open, turn off. Shell them all except 4-5 mussels and 4-5 clams which you will use to decorate; filter the cooking liquid. Beat the egg and the yolk with the filtered liquid, the cream and the parmesan. Brown the mussels in a pan, coated with new oil, and the diced squid for 1 minute, then add the mussels and shelled clams. Boil the tagliolini for 1-2 minutes, drain them in the pan with the mussels and add the beaten egg with the parmesan; mix quickly, distribute on plates, complete with the shellfish kept aside, a little parsley and a drizzle of raw oil and serve immediately.

SPAGHETTI WITH GARLIC, OIL AND CHILI PEPPER

Time 20 min

ingredients

Portions for 4 people

350 grams of spaghetti

3 fresh chillies

3 cloves of garlic

half onion

parsley

extra virgin olive oil

vinegar

salt

Preparation

For the spaghetti garlic, oil and chilli recipe, chop the fresh garlic. Peel the peppers and simmer them, covered, with the sliced onion and 30 g of vinegar for 10 minutes. Blend everything, make a sauce, pass it through a sieve and cook for 2 minutes to reduce it. Brown the chopped garlic in a pan with a few tablespoons of oil. Cook the spaghetti in boiling salted water, drain them and sauté them in a pan with the garlic. Serve them completely last with the chopped parsley and chopped garlic and the chilli sauce.

CRUDAIOLA SEDANINI

Time 15 min

ingredients

4 servings

300 g sedanini type pasta

8 courgette flowers

2 courgettes

2 firm tomatoes

parsley, basil, chives

salt and pepper

extra virgin olive oil

Preparation

For the recipe for raw celery, put a pan with the water for the pasta on the heat.

Salt it and, when it boils, add the celery. In the meantime, prepare the vegetables: cut the courgettes into quarters, lengthwise, and remove the central part with the seeds. Finally cut them into sticks, diagonally. Place them in a bowl with a little salt for 5 minutes. Cut the tomatoes into four segments, remove the seeds and also cut them into sticks. Pat the courgettes dry with kitchen paper, remove the water and mix with the tomatoes. Clean the courgette flowers, remove the pistil, rinse them and chop them in the bowl, adding them to the courgettes and tomatoes. Chop a sprig of parsley and some chives and season the vegetables with the chopped mixture, 4-5 tablespoons of oil and a little pepper. Drain the pasta and pour it into the vegetable bowl. Mix and complete with two basil leaves.

SALAD OF BUCKWHEAT, CANNELLINI BEANS AND COURGETTES

Time 45 min

ingredients

4 servings

300 g of boiled cannellini beans

250 g of trumpet courgettes

150 g of buckwheat

shallot, bay leaf

parsley, lemon

dry white wine

vegetable broth

extra virgin olive oil

salt and pepper

Preparation

Sauté half a shallot in 2 tablespoons of oil, then add the cannellini beans; flavor for 2-3 minutes, then pour in a large glass of white wine, let it evaporate, salt and add a bay leaf; after 15 minutes, add half a liter of vegetable broth and continue cooking for 10-15 minutes. Blend 100 g of cannellini beans with a spoonful of oil until you obtain a velvety cream. Keep the other cannellini beans aside. Cook the buckwheat in plenty of boiling vegetable broth for 17-18 minutes. Schoolboy.

Brown it in a pan with a drizzle of oil until it becomes crispy. Clean the Trombetta courgettes, cut them into quarters lengthwise and then cut them into lozenges. Cook them in a non-stick pan with a drizzle of oil and a sprig of chopped parsley for 3-4 minutes. Mix the cannellini bean cream with the buckwheat in a bowl, then add the courgettes, the remaining cannellini beans and complete with grated lemon zest, a few parsley leaves and pepper.

TESTAROLI WITH PESTO

FOR EVERYONE

Time 2 hours

ingredients

4 servings

180 g of 00 flour

80 g of buckwheat flour

80 g of rice flour, 60 g of pine nuts

60 g of green basil leaves

40 g of rice starch

30 g of macadamia nuts

a clove of garlic

grated cheese, red basil

salt and pepper

extra virgin olive oil

Preparation

Toast the coarsely chopped macadamia nuts in a pan and the pine nuts in another pan. Blend the green basil, the peeled and chopped garlic clove, 30 g of toasted pine nuts, 80 g of oil and a spoonful of grated cheese. Season with salt and pepper. For the Testaroli, mix the 00 flour with a whisk with 350 g of water and a pinch of salt until you obtain a fluid and homogeneous mixture. Leave to rest covered for an hour. Grease a cast iron pan (diameter 24 cm) well, heat it and then distribute a couple of ladles of the mixture. Cook it for 3 minutes, then turn it to the opposite side with the help of a spatula and continue cooking for another minute. Repeat the operation until the mixture is used up.

PASTA ALLA NORMA

Time 50 min

ingredients

4 servings

1 kg of tomatoes

400 g of aubergines

350 g of short celery-type pasta

150 g of salted ricotta

basil

half onion

extra virgin olive oil

peanut oil, salt

Preparation

For the pasta alla Norma recipe, coarsely chop the onion and sauté it in a saucepan with

3 tablespoons of extra virgin olive oil. Cut the tomatoes into large pieces. Prepare an aromatic bunch with about ten basil leaves. Add the bunch of basil to the saucepan and, after a minute, also the cherry tomatoes, add salt and cook for 25 minutes. Remove the basil for a couple of minutes before turning off the heat. Pass the tomato sauce through a food mill. Wash the aubergines and cut them into 3-4 mm thick slices; fry them in abundant hot peanut oil for 1-2 minutes. Cook the celery in abundant boiling salted water. Season them with tomato sauce and a drizzle of extra virgin olive oil, distribute them on plates and complete them with the fried aubergines, a few basil leaves and a generous grating of salted ricotta.

SALAD OF LITTLE RINGS, MOLLUSCS, CUCUMBERS AND MANGO

Time 1h 10min + 3h rest

ingredients

4 people

350 g of mussels

300 g clams

250 g of pasta such as anellini

200 g of clean medium-sized cuttlefish

150 g of cucumber

100 grams of mango

1 not too ripe tomato

shallot, parsley

white wine, garlic

pepper, basil

lemon, salt

extra virgin olive oil

Preparation

For the cannellini, shellfish, cucumber and mango salad recipe, soak the clams in cold salted water for at least 2 hours, changing the water three times; beat lightly to remove any damaged clams. Peel the cucumber, remove the seeds and cut it into 5 mm cubes; salt them and let them rest for 30 minutes, then squeeze out the water and dry them with kitchen paper. Place the mussels in a saucepan with 2-3 tablespoons of water, 2-3 tablespoons of wine, a sprig of parsley and 1 lightly crushed clove of garlic.

Cover and bring to the heat; once the shells have been opened, turn off and leave to cool with the lid on, then remove the shells. Keep the fruits immersed in the filtered cooking water, so that they do not dry out. Repeat the same procedure to open the clams. Place the whole cuttlefish in a saucepan with cold water, 1 slice of lemon, a sprig of parsley and 1 slice of shallot; cook for 5 minutes after boiling, turn off and leave to cool in the cooking water. Cut the cuttlefish into small pieces. Cut the tomato and mango into cubes. Mix the mango, tomatoes, cucumber, cuttlefish, mussels and shelled clams and season with a few spoonfuls of the previously filtered clam cooking water. Cover with cling film and leave to marinate for 1 hour in the fridge; finally season with salt. Boil the anelletti in boiling salted water for 7 minutes; remove them from the heat and leave them in the water for another 5 minutes; drain them, season them with a couple of tablespoons of oil, spread them on a tray and let them cool. Salt them and add them to the other ingredients, season with pepper and oil; scented with chopped basil leaves and finely chopped lemon zest.

COD PARMIGIANA

Time 50 min

ingredients

4 people

2 kg of purple aubergines

650 g desalted cod

200 g Provola

150 g of pitted olives

3 cans of cherry tomatoes

20 g of desalted salted capers

Grated Parmesan cheese

Peanut oil

00 flour, garlic, salt

extra virgin olive oil

Preparation

For the cod parmigiana recipe, prepare the sauce: in a pan, brown 1 clove of garlic in a thin layer of extra virgin olive oil, then add the olives, capers and cherry tomatoes; add salt and cook for about ten minutes. Cut the aubergines into slices lengthwise. Immerse in a bowl with cold water and ice for 10 minutes: the ice water will give compactness to the aubergines allowing them to be cut more easily after cooking without fraying. Flour the aubergines without letting them dry and fry them in boiling peanut oil; when they are golden, arrange them on kitchen paper. Blanch the cod in boiling unsalted water for

3-4 minutes, drain and, as soon as possible, flake; do this just before making the parmigiana to prevent the cod pieces from drying out. Assemble the parmigiana by alternating layers: on the bottom a layer of sauce, then the aubergines, followed by the pieces of cod and the provola cheese grated into large flakes; cover with a layer of sauce and aubergines; repeat the process until the ingredients are used up. Finally add a sprinkling of grated parmesan. Bake in a preheated oven at 180°C for about 20 minutes.

AROMATIC COLD SPAGHETTI

Time 20 min

ingredients

4 servings

500 g of spaghetti

200 grams of mozzarella

150 g of pitted olives

50 g of anchovy fillets in oil

8 radishes

fennel, basil

extra virgin olive oil

lemon, salt

Preparation

For the aromatic cold spaghetti recipe, chop a bunch of fennel and a sprig of basil and mix them with 150 g of oil, the grated zest of 1 lemon and the juice of half a fruit, the chopped anchovy fillets and a pinch of salt. if necessary. Peel the radishes and cut them into very thin slices; soak them in very cold water to make them crunchy. Cut the mozzarella into cubes. Boil the spaghetti for 7-8 minutes (they must remain al dente) and cool them immediately in cold water. Drain them and season them with the aromatic oil, radishes, mozzarella and olives; complete with fennel sprigs.

RIGATONI WITH FIVE TOMATOES

Time 1h

ingredients

4 servings

350 g rigatoni

200 g San Marzano tomatoes

180 g of cherry tomatoes

180 g of datterini cherry tomatoes

80 g of green tomato

50 g of yellow cherry tomatoes

30 g of carrots

30 g of onion

30 grams of celery

1 clove of garlic

tomato paste, thyme, basil

extra virgin olive oil, coarse salt

Preparation

For the five tomato rigatoni recipe, sauté the cherry tomatoes: blanch in boiling salted water for 45 seconds, drain them in a bowl with water and ice and peel them, keeping the peel aside. Then cook them in a pan over low heat with a drizzle of extra virgin olive oil, a sprig of thyme and 1/2 teaspoon of brown sugar, for about 40 minutes. Arrange the datterini tomatoes in a pan with the skins of the cherry tomatoes and let them dry in the oven at 140°C for about 40 minutes. In the meantime, prepare the tomato puree: dice the garlic, celery, carrot and onion and brown them in a pan with a drizzle of extra virgin olive oil.

extra virgin olive oil for 3 minutes over moderate heat. Add 2 teaspoons of tomato paste, a pinch of coarse salt and 1 teaspoon of brown sugar. Add the San Marzano tomatoes cut into coarse pieces and cook over low heat, with the lid on, for about twenty minutes; if necessary, add a ladle of boiling water. Finally pass through the food mill. Reduce the sauce in a saucepan for about ten minutes, adding a couple of basil leaves. Boil the rigatoni in abundant salted water, drain them al dente directly into the saucepan with the tomato puree and finish cooking by sautéing for a few minutes. Cut the green tomato and the yellow cherry tomatoes into 4 cubes and add them to the pasta with the cherry tomatoes, dried date tomatoes and the peels. Complete with basil and a drizzle of oil.

SPAGHETTI ALL'SCOGLIO

Time 1h 30min

ingredients

4 servings

320 grams of spaghetti

4 prawns, 4 scampi

2 calamari, 200 g of clams

200 g of mussels

a clove of garlic

a glass of white wine

a few spoonfuls of tomato puree

chopped parsley

extra virgin olive oil

salt, fresh pepper

Preparation

For the spaghetti, seafood recipe, clean the prawns and scampi, remove the casing and keep the heads. Brown the heads cut in half in a little oil, pour in half the wine and cover with cold water; leave to cook for at least an hour. Filter and reserve the shellfish broth. Chop the garlic, brown it in a little oil, add the clams and mussels and leave to open, adding the rest of the wine. Save the cooking liquid and quickly brown the prawns, scampi and squid, well cleaned and cut into small pieces. Add the tomato puree, the cooking juices from the clams and mussels, a little shellfish broth and cook for a few minutes. Cook the pasta in plenty of salted water, drain it and finish cooking in the sauce, add the chopped fresh chilli, parsley, clams and mussels. Stir in a little oil and serve.

RISOTTO AND PEAS, SCAMPI AND LEMON

Time 45 minutes

ingredients

4 servings

400 g of fresh peas in pods

350 g of Carnaroli rice

12 pieces of scampi

1 piece of celery stalk

1 carrot

1 shallot, 1 lemon

dry white wine, thyme

extra virgin olive oil

coarse salt

Preparation

For the risotto with peas, scampi and lemon recipe, shell the peas and collect them little by little in a bowl of cold water; keep the pods aside. Shell the prawns: remove the heads; then, holding the tails between your fingers, use scissors to make a long cut in the center between the legs. Turn the tail and cut it on the back in the same way. Finally, widen the carapace and remove the tail by pulling it gently, keeping the heads and shells. Prepare the broth: cut the celery, carrot and 1/2 shallot in half; brown them in a large pan in a thin layer of extra virgin olive oil; after 5 minutes add the pods and fry them for 5 minutes;

then add 1 liter of water and the scampi shells; cook over a very moderate heat for 20 minutes, making sure it never reaches the boil. Remove the shells; coarsely blend the broth and vegetables and finally filter the broth through a sieve. Toast the rice in a saucepan with a drizzle of oil for a couple of minutes, add 1/2 chopped shallot and deglaze with 1/2 glass of white wine; when the wine has evaporated, cook the rice for 12-13 minutes, wetting it from time to time with a ladle of broth; then add the peas and a pinch of coarse salt and finish cooking in another 3-4 minutes. At the end add a few leaves of thyme, and the juice obtained by crushing the scampi heads directly into the risotto. Complete with the scampi tails, diced or whole, the grated lemon zest and serve.

ORECCHIETTE WITH TOMATO

Time 45 minutes

ingredients

6 servings

1 kg of ripe tomatoes

400 g of re-milled semolina

Grain semolina

1 clove of garlic

salt, hard ricotta, basil

extra virgin olive oil

Preparation

Cut the tomatoes with a cross cut; blanch them in water for 30 seconds, drain them, peel them and cut them into small pieces, removing the seeds. Cook them in a pan with 3 tablespoons of oil and the garlic clove with the peel for 15-20 minutes; remove the garlic and salt.

For the orecchiette Knead the semolina with about 220 g of warm salted water, until you obtain a dough with a consistency similar to that of bread: the exact quantity of water to mix depends on the quality of the semolina. Divide the dough into loaves (ø approximately cm) and divide them into 1 cm long pieces. Drag each piece onto the well-floured work surface (the ideal is to use a wooden pastry board) with a finger or a knife with a rounded tip, then turn it over giving the classic shape of the ears. Cook the orecchiette in plenty of salted water; drain them when they float to the surface and season them with the tomato sauce. Complete with plenty of grated ricotta, basil leaves and serve.

CREAM OF PEAS WITH TOMATOES AND RASPBERRY SAUCE

Time 1h

ingredients

4 people

1.3 kg of fresh peas

500 g of potatoes

200 g of datterini cherry tomatoes

125 g of raspberries

10 g of brown sugar, half an onion

extra virgin olive oil

salt and pepper

Preparation

Cut the dates into small pieces and place them in a saucepan with a drizzle of oil. Add 100 g of raspberries and the brown sugar.

Add salt and pepper and cook for 10-12 minutes. Blend everything with the immersion blender and filter until you obtain a smooth sauce. Shell 1 kg of peas. Peel the potatoes and cut them into slices. Chop the onion and sauté it in a saucepan with a drizzle of oil for 3-4 minutes. Add the potatoes and cover them with water, salt and pepper; cook for about 20 minutes. Add the shelled peas and cook for another 3-4 minutes. Blend the pods with as much water as you need to make a smoothie. Pass it through a sieve to obtain 200 g of juice. Add it to the saucepan and stir for 1-2 minutes. Blend everything with the immersion blender into a cream that is not too smooth. Serve with the sauce, completing with some raspberries and the remaining raw, shelled peas.

RISOTTO WITH CHICKEN WINGS AND CARROT BUTTER

Time 1h 10min

+ 30 minutes of rest

ingredients

4 people

For Carrot Butter

200 g of carrots

70 g of butter, salt

320 g of Carnaroli rice

4 chicken wings

1/2 shallot

black peppercorns

lemon, rosemary

marjoram, parsley

dry white wine

Grated Parmesan cheese

Preparation

Peel the carrots and cut them into slices. Place them in a saucepan with the butter, 200 g of water and a pinch of salt. Let them simmer for about 20 minutes until the water has completely evaporated. Blend the carrots and spread the cream obtained on a baking tray to cool. Then collect it in a bowl and place it in the refrigerator for at least 30 minutes. Even better if you prepare this butter the day before. Rinse the wings and place them in a saucepan with 1.3 liters of water, 200 g of white wine, 6-7 peppercorns, a lemon zest, a sprig of rosemary, marjoram and parsley. Bring to the boil and cook over medium heat for about 45 minutes. Remove the fins and filter the broth. Chop the shallot and sauté it in a saucepan with a small knob of butter. Toast the rice, deglaze it with 1/2 glass of wine, then add the fine broth. Cook by adding the broth little by little, in about 16 minutes. Finally, stir in the carrot butter and 2 tablespoons of grated parmesan. Remove the pulp from the wings, chop the meat and serve with the risotto and grated carrots to taste.

MIXED PASTA AND MUSSELS WITH LIME AND CHILI PEPPER

Time 30 min

ingredients

4 people

2 kg of cleaned mussels

320 g of mixed short pasta

100g of grated pecorino

2 cloves of garlic, 1 lime

chili

dry white wine

extra virgin olive oil

salt and pepper

Preparation

For the mixed pasta and mussels with lime and chilli pepper recipe, clean and rinse the mussels; Place them in a pan with 3 tablespoons of oil, heat with the peeled garlic and 1 chopped chilli pepper. Wet them with a splash of white wine, cover them and cook for about 5-6 minutes, until the shells have opened. Drain the mussels and filter their sauce. Rinse the pan. Boil the pasta in boiling salted water for 2 minutes less than the indicated cooking time. In the meantime, shell the mussels, leaving a dozen in the half shell, to decorate the dishes. Pour 2-3 ladles of mussel sauce into the pan and bring back to the boil. Add the drained pasta and finish cooking, adding the shelled mussels at the end. Mixed with the pecorino and served completing with the mussels in half shell, a grind of pepper and the grated zest of the lime.

**RISOTTO AND PRAWNS
WITH PEPPER SAUCE**

Time 1h

ingredients

4 servings

350 g Vialone nano rice

12 shrimp

4 red peppers

a shallot

toasted hazelnuts

pickled capers

extra virgin olive oil, salt

Preparation

Place the peppers on a baking tray lined with baking paper and cook them at 240°C for 25-30 minutes; let them cool, peel them and cut them

fillets, removing the seeds. Blend in the sauce, keeping aside a couple of fillets that you will use, chopped, as a garnish for the dish. Peel the shallot and chop it. Heat the rice in a saucepan with a generous pinch of salt; when it is hot to the touch, add the shallot, mix, pour a ladle of hot water and cook for 8-10 minutes, adding more water if necessary (it must be dry at the end). Spread out on a baking tray and let it cool. Shell the prawns and sear them in a pan with a drizzle of oil and a pinch of salt for a minute. Coarsely chop a dozen hazelnuts and 2 tablespoons of capers. Shell the rice, add it to the pepper sauce, place the prawns on top and garnish with chopped hazelnuts and capers, pieces of pepper and, if desired, pickled caper leaves and marjoram.

SPAGHETTI WITH GUITAR WITH SPOTLIGHTS

Time 1h

ingredients

4 servings

500 g of tomato puree

300 g minced beef pulp

200 g of 0 flour

200 g of regrind

whole wheat flour

60 g of grated cheese

40 g of breadcrumbs

4 eggs, sugar, nutmeg

milk, garlic, white onion

extra virgin olive oil

salt and pepper

Preparation

Mix the two flours, add them to the eggs and let the mixture rest, covered, for 30 minutes. Flour the work surface and roll out the dough until it is 2 mm thick. Roll out the dough on the guitar and press it well against the strings with the help of a rolling pin, thus obtaining spaghetti. Spread out on a tray, dusting with a little durum wheat flour to prevent them from sticking. In a saucepan, fry half a chopped onion and a crushed garlic clove with the peel in 3 tablespoons of oil for 2-3 minutes. Add the tomato puree, a glass of water, salt and a pinch of sugar and continue cooking for 25-30 minutes.

Soak the breadcrumbs in 5 tablespoons of milk, squeeze it well and add it to the minced meat and grated cheese; add a generous grating of nutmeg, salt and pepper and mix well. Form balls the size of olives and cook, little by little, in a large pan with 4 tablespoons of hot oil for 1-2, stirring to roast them evenly. Season the balls with half the tomato sauce. Cook the spaghetti alla guitar in abundant boiling salted water for 4-5 minutes; drain them al dente and season them in a pan with the remaining tomato sauce. Arrange the spaghetti on plates, garnish with the balls and season to taste with grated pecorino and pepper.

SPRUCE RISOTTO

Time 40 min

ingredients

4 people

320 g of Carnaroli rice

300 g fir sprigs

fresh red (Picea abies)

100 g parmesan

50 g of fresh butter

20 g of lemon juice

extra virgin olive oil

salt

Preparation

For the spruce risotto recipe, bring 2 liters of water to the boil and immerse half the spruce sprigs in it, boil them for 8-10 minutes, then turn off and leave to infuse to obtain a broth. Chop the rest of the sprigs and extract the juice with an extractor. It will be a little difficult to extract due to the woodier part, but by passing it several times and adding about 300 g of water, you will obtain a smooth juice. Alternatively, blend just the needles with an immersion blender adding 300g of water and then strain through a fine sieve lined with cheesecloth. Keep the residues aside, spread them on a baking tray lined with baking paper and dry them in the oven in the oven for 4-5 hours at 45°C or in the dehydrator: you can use them to flavor a pizza or to prepare an aromatic salt. Heat a saucepan with a drizzle of oil, pour in the rice, and toast it with a pinch of salt for at least 1-2 minutes: when the grains are hot it is time to start pouring in the fir broth, alternating it a little at a time with the extract (keep aside a couple of spoonfuls to finish at the end). Cook the rice for 13-14 minutes, stirring constantly, then remove from the heat and stir in the butter, grated parmesan and a few drops of lemon juice. Top with a few drops of spruce extract and serve immediately.

SEMOLINA FUNNELS WITH RAGU

Time 55 min

ingredients

4 people

400 g regrind

durum wheat flour

300 g of tomato puree

250 g of minced beef pulp

150 g of white wine

100 g of chopped raw ham

50 g of seed oil

2 stalks of celery

2 carrots, 2 onions

salt and pepper

Preparation

For the recipe for semolina funnels with ragù, mix the semolina with 400 g of water at room temperature for 10 minutes. Leave to rest for 20 minutes, then roll out the dough with a rolling pin or pasta machine to a thickness of 2 mm. Using a pastry cutter or a small glass (ø 4 cm), cut out discs. Take them in your hand and pinch the two ends between your index finger and thumb, leaving a small hole to create a sort of small funnel. Let dry. Finely chop the celery, carrots and onions and fry them in vegetable oil, then add the minced meat and ham.

Brown for a few minutes, add the white wine and let them dry. Add the tomato puree, 500 g of water and plenty of pepper. As soon as the mixture comes to the boil, lower the heat and cook covered, over low heat, for 20 minutes. Add salt only at the end of cooking: Cook the funnels in plenty of salted water, drain them, season them with the ragù and serve hot.

SPAGHETTI WITH SHRIMPS AND COCONUT

Time 10 min

ingredients

4 servings

250 grams of spaghetti

50 g of butter

30g grated coconut

16 pieces of shrimp

extra virgin olive oil

herbs and flowers

salt

Preparation

For the shrimp and coconut spaghetti recipe, cook the spaghetti for 5 minutes in boiling salted water. In the meantime, remove the prawn heads and crush them in a sieve, recovering the juice. Shell the tails and season them with a drizzle of oil. Melt the butter in a pan and emulsify it with a ladle of pasta cooking water. Drain the spaghetti and sauté them in the pan with the butter. Arrange them on plates and season them with prawn juice, raw prawns, grated coconut and aromatic herbs.

STUFFED MACARONI TIMBALE

Time 1h 20 min

Ingredients, 4 people

300 g of minced veal pulp

250 g of macaroni

30 g of grated pecorino cheese

10 thin slices of Emmental

3 eggs, 1 onion

Grated Parmesan cheese

butter, bay leaf

tomato paste, vegetable broth

extra virgin olive oil, salt and pepper

Preparation

For the stuffed macaroni timbale recipe, prepare the ragù as in the traditional pan:

Brown the onion, combine the meat with salt and pepper, add the wine, then add 1 tablespoon of concentrate, the broth and cook for 1 hour. Boil the macaroni, drain them 2 minutes before the end of cooking and season them with 20 g of butter. Beat the eggs with the pecorino, salt, pepper and 2 tablespoons of broth. Chop the ragù in the cutter to make it finer, and mix it with a third of the egg mixture. Scoop it into a pastry bag with an opening as wide as a macaroni. Butter 2 molds (ø 12 cm) and make a layer of cheese slices, then add 2 tablespoons of egg mixture. Arrange the macaroni vertically in the moulds, distribute the remaining egg mixture, then fill the macaroni with the ragù. Sprinkle with parmesan and bake at 190°C for 10-15 minutes.

BUCATINI WITH RICOTTA, LEMON AND CAPERS

Time 10 min

ingredients

4 servings

350 g bucatini

250 g of fresh ricotta

50 g of sesame breadsticks

pickled capers

lemongrass

extra virgin olive oil

Lemon

salt and pepper

Preparation

For the bucatini recipe with ricotta, lemon and capers, cook the pasta in boiling salted water. Crumble half the ricotta in a pan with 3 tablespoons of oil, pepper and 1 ladle of pasta cooking water. Add 2 tablespoons of drained capers and the grated zest of 1 lemon. Break the sesame breadsticks into pieces. Drain the pasta and mix it in the pan with the ricotta. Serve by adding the remaining ricotta, crumbled breadsticks, more grated lemon zest, a drizzle of raw oil and lemongrass leaves.

HALF PENNE WITH LEMON, MUSTARD AND ANCHOVIES

Time 15 min

ingredients

4 servings

350 g of half penne

50 g of butter

6 anchovy fillets

2 teaspoons of mustard

a lemon

a spoonful of desalted capers

salt and pepper

Preparation

For the recipe for mezze penne with lemon, mustard and anchovies, cook the pasta in boiling salted water. In the meantime, prepare the mustard, butter, grated zest of half a lemon, 4 chopped anchovies and ground pepper in a bowl. Drain the pasta, pour it into the bowl and mix. Prepare the dishes and add the remaining chopped anchovies, capers and pieces of lemon pulp. Garnish as desired: we added some dill leaves and a little chilli.

NETTLE GNOCCHI WITH TOMATO

Time 1h

ingredients

4 servings

500 g of 0 flour

400 g of nettles

350 g of tomato puree

4 eggs, sage, basil, salt and pepper

extra virgin olive oil

Preparation

For the tomato nettle gnocchi recipe, cook the tomato puree over a low heat with a couple of spoons of oil and a pinch of salt. Turn off after 18-20 minutes, add a generous sprig of basil leaves and some sage leaves, cover and leave to infuse for 5 minutes. For the gnocchi, peel the nettles, blanch them in boiling salted water for 1 minute, drain them and squeeze them well: depending on how much you squeeze them you will obtain a more or less moist mixture. Blend with an immersion blender, then mix them with the flour, eggs and a pinch of salt, and you will obtain a soft dough. Divide it into loaves of a couple of centimeters in diameter; cut them into 2cm pieces and shape the gnocchi by rubbing them on the tines of the fork. Distribute them on the floured work surface. Boil the gnocchi in abundant boiling salted water for 10-12 minutes. Drain and season with tomato puree and freshly ground pepper. Decorate as desired with sage leaves.

RIGATONI WITH PEPPERS, SHRIMP AND HAZELNUTS

Time 1h

ingredients

6 servings

500 g giant rigatoni

100 g of grated pecorino

100 g of latte macchiato

50 g of toasted hazelnuts

12 prawn tails

3 large red peppers

extra virgin olive oil

mind, sale

Preparation

Arrange the peppers on a baking tray lined with baking paper and bake at 250°C for about 30 minutes. Remove E from the oven, let them cool, then peel them, remove the seeds and blend 2/3 with a little salt. Keep the cream warm. For the pecorino cream, bring the milk to the boil, remove it from the heat, add the pecorino and mix well until it has completely dissolved; finally blend until you obtain a smooth cream. Keep him warm. Shell the prawn tails, remove the casing and cut them into pieces. Cut the rest of the peppers into squares. For the pasta, boil the rigatoni in boiling salted water, drain and season with a drizzle of oil, the squares of pepper and pieces of prawns. Distribute the two creams on the plates, arrange the pasta, mix delicately and add the chopped hazelnuts and mint leaves.

PARSLEY RISOTTO WITH PUMPKIN FLOWERS MUSSELS AND CLAMS

Time 1h 50min

ingredients

4 servings

300 g of Carnaroli rice

300 g clams

300 g of cleaned mussels

150 g of parsley

8 courgette flowers

1 clove of garlic

dry white wine

lemon, vegetable broth

salt and pepper

extra virgin olive oil

Preparation

For the parsley risotto with mussels and clams recipe, drain the clams in salted water for 1 hour, changing the water after 30 minutes. Open the clams and mussels together in a saucepan with a drizzle of oil, ground pepper and 1 clove of garlic. Strain their cooking liquid into a fine sieve lined with kitchen paper. Shell the mussels and clams, keeping some of the prettiest shells aside for garnish.

Clean the parsley, blanch the leaves in salted water for a couple of minutes, drain them, squeeze them lightly and blend until you obtain a cream. Toast the rice in a saucepan greased with a drizzle of oil and a good pinch of salt for 1 minute; Add half a glass of wine and cook for 15-17 minutes, wetting it occasionally with 1 ladle of vegetable broth and, finally, with 1 ladle of shell liquid. Stir the risotto with 3 tablespoons of oil and the parsley cream; add 4 courgette flowers cut into strips. Distribute the rice on the plates, complete with all the mussels and clams, the remaining courgette flower petals and the grated lemon zest.

PENNE WITH ASPARAGUS, BUTTER AND ALMONDS

Time 30 min

ingredients

4 servings

850 g of asparagus

350 g of mezze penne rigate

70 g of flaked almonds

30 g of butter

marjoram, salt

Preparation

For the asparagus, butter and almond penne recipe, clean the asparagus by removing the fibrous peel with a potato peeler. Drain them for 4-5 minutes in boiling water.

Cool in water and ice, then cut the stems into pieces, keeping the tips intact. Melt the butter in a large skillet; add the almonds, sauté them for 30 seconds, then add the asparagus rolls and the chopped marjoram. Boil the penne, drain them al dente and add them to the pan with the sauce. Sauté everything for 1-2 minutes, adding, if necessary, a few tablespoons of cooking water. Finally, add suggestions. Serve the pasta piping hot, topped with grated parmesan if desired.

CARBONARA" WITH CUTTLEFISH, ASPARAGUS AND SPECK

Time 40 min

ingredients

4 people

800 g of white asparagus

200 g of cleaned cuttlefish

8 slices of speck

2 egg yolks

chili pepper, lemon

vegetable broth

extra virgin olive oil

seed oil, dill, salt

Preparation

Prepare a spicy mayonnaise: whip the 2 egg yolks by slowly adding 150 g of extra virgin olive oil, alternating with 150 g of seed oil. Transfer the mayonnaise into a bowl, add 20 ml of vegetable broth, a splash of lemon juice and a pinch of chopped chilli pepper, mix well and season with salt. Heat a pan with plenty of seed oil and fry the slices of speck cut in half until they are crispy. Drain them on kitchen paper and break half into crumbs, rubbing them on a sheet of kitchen paper to remove the grease well; keep the other 8 pieces aside for the final garnish. Brown the cuttlefish in extra virgin olive oil over high heat with a pinch of chilli for 1 minute;

add a splash of lemon juice and a pinch of salt and turn off. Let them cool and cut them into thin strips. Clean the asparagus, remove the final part of the stem and first slice thinly lengthwise with a mandolin or potato peeler and then into vertical strips, making them similar to spaghetti. Boil them in boiling salted water for 3 minutes. Drain them on absorbent paper. Mix the cuttlefish and asparagus and season them with the mayonnaise, keeping a few spoons aside; add salt if necessary. Distribute the carbonara on the plates, complete with the speck crumbs, the dill leaves and the remaining mayonnaise; garnish each dish with slices of speck and bring to the table and serve.

FETTUCCINE AND SCAMPI ON ASPARAGUS CREAM

Duration 50 min

ingredients

4 servings

400 g of fresh fettuccine

200 g of cucumbers

200 g of fresh shelled peas

120 g of new spinach

12 scampi

11 green asparagus

1 pc lime, vegetable broth

extra virgin olive oil

sale, pepper

Preparation

For the fettuccine and scampi recipe on asparagus cream, peel the cucumbers, keep the peel aside and cut them into chunks. Marina Teli with 2 tablespoons of oil, a pinch of salt, a grind of pepper and the juice of 1/2 lime for 30 minutes. Blanch the cucumber peels for a few seconds in boiling salted water; drain them and, in the same water, blanch the peas for 2-3 minutes. Clean the asparagus and cook 3 with 1 glass of broth for 5 minutes; Season with salt and blend to obtain a cream. Cut the remaining asparagus lengthwise into thin sticks. Shell the scampi, remove the dark casing and brown them in a greased pan with a drizzle of oil, for 30 seconds; salt and pepper and free the pan. Boil the fettuccine in plenty of salted water until they float to the surface. In the meantime, in the same pan as the scampi, cook the spinach, the asparagus sticks and the cucumber peels with the juice of 1/2 lime, 2 tablespoons of the fettuccine cooking water, a pinch of salt and a grind of pepper to 2-3 minutes. Season the fettuccine with the asparagus cream, and distribute on the plates, complete with the scampi, all the vegetables, the peas, the pieces of marinated cucumber and the grated lime zest.

RECIPES
SECOND DISHES

FISH STEWAND ZUCCHINI CREAM WITH SCAPECE

Time 1h 30min

ingredients

4 people

The courgette cream

250g chicken stock

5 courgettes

1/2 shallot

potatoes, mint

White wine vinegar

extra virgin olive oil

salt and pepper, the stew

100 g of red mullet fillets

100 g of tuna fillet

100 g of sea bass fillet, 4 scallops, 4 prawns

4 scampi, 4 clams, 4 mussels

1 clove of garlic, parsley, salt

extra virgin olive oil

Preparation

Peel the courgettes, remove the part with the seeds and cut them into pieces. In a saucepan, fry the chopped shallot and a piece of finely chopped potato, add the courgettes and let them flavour. Douse them with a splash of vinegar, then add the hot chicken broth. Season with leaves of a few minutes and cook for 20 minutes. Blend everything, adding salt and pepper and slowly adding 2-3 tablespoons of oil (for a greener sauce, peel the courgettes and blanch the peels in boiling salted water; proceed with the recipe, cutting the peeled courgettes into cubes. When it's time to blend to obtain the sauce, add the blanched peels (if you want it very velvety, pass it through a sieve). Place the peeled garlic in a saucepan with a drizzle of oil and a little parsley. When the oil is hot, add the mussels and cover. Wet with a drop of water and cover again. Remove the mussels from the pan as soon as they open. Repeat the operation with the clams. Clean all the fish and cut them into small pieces. Shelled prawns, scampi and scallops. Drizzle them with a drizzle of oil and drain them for 3-4 minutes in a hot pan, sprinkled with a pinch of salt. Serve fish, molluscs and crustaceans on the.

FISH MEATLOAF WITH BROCCOLI, AROMATIC HERBS

Time 1h

ingredients

6-8 people

580 g of cleaned cod fillet

120 g of broccoli tufts

4 egg whites

coriander berries, green pepper

dill, chives, salt

Preparation

For the fish meatloaf with broccoli and aromatic herbs recipe, blanch the broccoli tufts in boiling salted water for 1 minute and drain them.

Clean the cod from any remaining bones, cut it into small pieces and add the egg whites and a pinch of salt. Blend everything until you obtain a slightly sticky mass. Flavored with ground coriander and green pepper. Add the broccoli tufts to the mixture, after having dabbed them with kitchen paper, to dry them a little. Also, add a sprig of chopped dill along with some chives. Spread the mixture on a layer of overlapping sheets of foil suitable for cooking. Roll it up with the help of the film until you obtain a sausage. Tie it at the ends with kitchen string and steam the meatloaf for 45 minutes. Accompanied to taste with a soft polenta, which you can prepare by cooking 50 g of yellow polenta flour in 500 g of boiling fish broth. Then mix with butter, salt and pepper and coriander, the same herbs used for the meatloaf.

PERCH AND TAPIOCA CUTTLET

Time 40 min

ingredients

6 people servings

6 perch fillets

300 grams of tomatoes

120 g tapioca pearls

corn flour

egg white

tomato concentrate

basil salt

Peanut oil

Preparation

For the perch and tapioca cutlet recipe, cut the cherry tomatoes into small pieces and blend them. Collect the pulp in a sieve lined with a cloth, place it on a container, and let it drain until you obtain 100 g of tomato water. Cook the tapioca in 300 g of boiling salted water. When the tapioca pearls begin to swell and become slightly transparent, add the tomato water and cook for 15-20 minutes. In the meantime, bread the fish fillets, dipping in the corn flour, then in 1 beaten egg white and again in the corn flour. Fry them in hot peanut oil for 2 minutes per side. Mix the pureed tomato pulp with 1 tablespoon of concentrate, obtaining a sauce. Serve the fried fillets in the tapioca soup and complete with tomato sauce and fresh basil leaves.

FLES WITH PORCINI AND POTATOES

Time 1h

ingredients

6 servings

6 small yellow potatoes

150 g of porcini mushrooms

30 g parmesan

2 pieces of shallots, butter

bay leaves, marjoram

tasty, wise

rosemary, red wine

tomato concentrate

extra virgin olive oil

salt and pepper

Preparation

For the potato flan recipe, peel the potatoes and wash them in a bowl until the water runs clear, to remove some of the starch. Cut the potatoes into regular slices 3-4 mm thick. Massage with a drizzle of oil, spread on a baking tray lined with baking paper and lightly salt them. Clean the porcini mushrooms, cut them into regular slices, distribute them in the pan with the potatoes and season them with a drizzle of oil. Bake at 220°C for 15 minutes. Butter 6 muffin molds (ø 7 cm) and line the bottom with 6 discs of baking paper, which should also be buttered. Finely chop a sprig of marjoram, savory, and a sprig of rosemary and mix in the grated parmesan. Remove the potatoes and porcini mushrooms from the oven and assemble each flan by distributing a a layer of potatoes, one of parmesan with herbs, and one of porcini mushrooms in each mould, repeat the three layers and finish with parmesan and a knob of butter; bake at 180-190°C for about ten minutes. Prepare the sauce: peel the shallot, cut it in half and brown it in a saucepan with a knob of butter, a sprig of sage, a couple of bay leaves, a pinch of salt and a grind of pepper. When the shallot begins to sizzle, add 1 glass of red wine and let it evaporate; add 1 teaspoon of tomato paste and cook for 10 minutes; finally remove the aromatic herbs and blend until you obtain a smooth and homogeneous sauce. Serve the flans with the sauce; accompanied to taste with porcini mushrooms sautéed in a pan with a knob of butter.

PORK SALTIMBOCCA WITH AUBERGINE CREAM

Time 1h

ingredients

4 people

600 g1 violet aubergine

450g 4 slices of real pork

120 g of breadcrumbs

30 g of fennel

parsley, basil

extra virgin olive oil

garlic salt

Preparation

For the recipe for pork saltimbocca with aubergine cream, chop the fennel and finely chop the stems as well. Heat 4 tablespoons of oil in a large pan with 1 clove of garlic in its peel; add the chopped fennel, mix and cook for 1 minute, then remove the garlic, season with salt and add the breadcrumbs. Leave to flavor on the heat for another 30 seconds, then turn off the heat and leave to cool. Beat the slices of meat, reducing them to a thickness of 3-4 mm; distribute 1 tablespoon of fennel-flavoured bread on half of each slice, then close them in a wallet. Spread a little more breadcrumbs on the surface of the saltimbocca, close them with a toothpick and season them with a drizzle of oil. Cook them on a hot grill for 8-9 minutes, turn them over and continue cooking for another 5-6 minutes, adding salt. Cut the aubergine in half and cut it into a lozenge shape cut it, oil it well and cook it in a very hot non-stick pan over a moderate heat, with a lid, for 10-12 minutes, then turn the two halves and continue cooking for another 10 minutes. until the pulp is soft (check with the tip of a knife). Turn off and leave to cool with the pan covered. Remove the pulp from the aubergine halves and blend the pulp with an immersion blender, adding the water released into the pan during cooking, 1 tablespoon of chopped parsley, a few torn basil leaves, a pinch of salt, 1 clove of garlic and 2 tablespoons of oil. Serve the saltimbocca, even at room temperature, with the aubergine puree, accompanying, if desired, with a salad of cherry tomatoes, basil and fennel.

CHICKEN STEW, VEAL, CHAMPIGNON MUSHROOMS

Time 1h

ingredients

8 servings

400 g of chicken breast

400 g of megatello or veal tip

250 g of champignon mushrooms

240 g of boiled cannellini beans

two stalks of white celery

an onion, white wine

cumin seeds

cinnamon powder

fennel seeds

fresh fennel, pepper

Nutmeg powder

extra virgin olive oil

salt and pepper

Preparation

For the chicken, veal and mushroom stew recipe, cut the chicken breast and veal into cubes of approximately 2 cm. Peel the celery and onion, cut them into small cubes, and brown them for 6-7 minutes with a drizzle of oil in a large pan, which will then contain everything else. Clean the champignon mushrooms, remove the stems and earthy residues, wash them briefly and slice them; add them to the pan with the onion and celery together with a pinch of salt and continue cooking for 10 minutes. Brown the meat cubes in a pan with a drizzle of oil and a pinch of salt for about 10 minutes:

to facilitate browning, collect any liquid
released; pour it into the pan with the
mushrooms to flavor them. Wet the meat
with 1/2 glass of wine and let it evaporate for
1 minute. Transfer everything to the pot with
the mushrooms, cover with water, add a
pinch of all the spices (dosing to taste), salt
and pepper, and cook gently for another 20
minutes, adding the drained cannellini beans
at the end. Distribute the stew on plates,
complete with the chopped fresh fennel and
slices of chilli, then serve.

SEABASS AND COURGETTE SKEWERS

Time 50 min

ingredients

4 people

600 g of sea bass fillets

350 g 1 large courgette

70 g of bread for sandwiches

lemon, garlic

Pepper

fresh chili pepper

Grana Padano Dop

chopped parsley

extra virgin olive oil

salt and pepper

Preparation

For the recipe for sea bass and courgette skewers, scale the sea bass fillets, trim them on the belly side and remove any bones. Cut the fillets into 4 lozenges from each and season them with a drizzle of oil. Blend the bread, without the edges, with 1 teaspoon of grated lemon zest, 1 tablespoon of grated parmesan, 1 tablespoon of chopped parsley, a pinch of salt, a grind of pepper and 1 tablespoon of oil. Cut the courgettes into four segments lengthwise and remove the central seeds; then cut each segment into 5 parts. Pass the sea bass lozenges in the breadcrumbs. Prepare the skewers by alternating the fish and courgettes on the skewer, so as to have 6 pieces of sea bass and 5 courgettes on each skewer, tightly pressed together. Place the skewers in a tray keeping them close together; Spread a little more breadcrumbs on top, then turn them over and distribute the remaining breadcrumbs, pressing with your hands to make them adhere well. Cook the skewers on a hot plate for 3 minutes, turn them over and continue cooking for another 3 minutes. Prepare a dressing by heating 2 tablespoons of oil with 2-3 cloves of garlic; add 1 tablespoon of chopped parsley, 1/2 tablespoon of diced pepper and a few slices of chili pepper, mix to flavor, turn off and leave to cool. Distribute the seasoning on the skewers and serve.

SLICET OF SALMON E MUSTARD SOUR CREAM

Time 35 min

ingredients

6 people servings

600 g of salmon fillet

200 grams of cream

wheat mustard

6 g of slices of homemade bread

Marjoram

cucumber, lemon

caper leaves

extra virgin olive oil

salt pink peppercorns

Preparation

For the salmon steak and mustard sour cream recipe, grease the slices of bread with a drizzle of oil, salt them and toast them in the pan for a couple of minutes on each side. Lay out a sheet of aluminum foil, place a sheet of baking paper on top and finally arrange the salmon steak. Season with the juice of 1/2 lemon, pink pepper, marjoram and 5-6 caper leaves. Close the foil and bake at 200°C for about 15 minutes. Whip the cream with a hand whisk with a pinch of salt, 1 teaspoon of lemon juice and 1 tablespoon of grain mustard. Serve the salmon with toasted bread, sour cream and cucumber slices.

OCTOPUS IN SALAD

Time 1h 30min

+ 30 minutes of marination

ingredients

4 people

600 g 1 fresh octopus

1 onion

1 stalk of celery

1 carrot, vinegar

1 clove of garlic

extra virgin olive oil

salt and pepper

cherry tomatoes

Preparation

For the traditional octopus salad recipe, bring a pot of water with the whole onion, celery and carrot to a boil. When it boils, dip the octopus and remove it immediately afterwards; repeat the operation 3-4 times, to curl the tentacles; then immerse it completely and let it cook for 40 minutes. Turn off and let the octopus cool in its water. Drain it and cut it into small pieces, keeping some of the most beautiful curls. Season it with 3 tablespoons of vinegar and the peeled, cored and chopped garlic clove. Leave to marinate for 30 minutes. Finally season it with oil, salt, pepper and chopped parsley. Accompany it, if you like, with some cherry tomatoes cut into wedges.

MONKFISH

AND RED GRAPES

Time 1h 20min

ingredients

6 people servings

1.5kg monkfish slice

200 grams of bacon

smoked in thin slices

500 g of red grapes

dry white wine

Thyme, butter

salt, pepper, sage

Preparation

For the monkfish and red grapes recipe, debone the fish steak by making an incision along the central bone, then remove it. Wrap the boneless steak in the bacon slices, overlapping them slightly; place the monkfish in a baking dish or baking dish, flavor with a sprig of sage, salt and pepper and cook at 180°C in a convection oven for about 30 minutes. Then wash the grapes, add them to the pan with 1/2 glass of white wine and continue cooking for another ten minutes. If you want to further check the cooking, use a probe thermometer to measure the core temperature: it must have reached 64°C. Transfer the monkfish to a serving plate, cover it with aluminum foil and let it rest for a few minutes. Bring the pan with the cooking liquid and grapes to the heat. Allow the sauce to reduce slightly, add a knob of butter and emulsify. Serve the monkfish steaks with the sauce and complete with a few sage leaves and a little thyme.

THREE COLORED ONIONS WITH CHICKPEAS, BREAD AND DRIED FRUIT

Time 1h 30min

ingredients

4 people

200 g of boiled chickpeas

60 g of wholemeal bread

30 g of pine nuts

30 g of pistachios

30 dried tomatoes in oil

2 red onions

2 copper onions

2 white onions

extra virgin olive oil

salt, pepper, bay leaf

Preparation

For the recipe of tricolor onions with chickpeas, bread and dried fruit, boil the onions in their skins in boiling salted water for 20 minutes, then drain them. Cut the caps and empty. Chop all the pulp obtained and sauté it in a pan with 3-4 tablespoons of oil and the diced bread for a couple of minutes. Also add the drained chickpeas, 2 bay leaves, salt and pepper and cook for 3-4 minutes. Also add the pine nuts and pistachios and cook for another 2 minutes.

Turn off and blend everything in the cutter, shaking it, so as to obtain a coarse filling. Add 2 more tablespoons of oil and season with salt and pepper. Stuff the onions with the filling, and also add the cherry tomatoes, alternating with the filling. Grease with a drizzle of oil and bake the onions together with the caps at 180°C for 30-40 minutes.

TUNA ESCALOP E
PINK GRAPEFRUIT

Time 35 min

ingredients

4 people servings

4 tuna steaks weighing 150 g

3 pink grapefruits

extra virgin olive oil

salt

1 slice of bread

pistachios

Sesame seeds

Preparation

For the tuna and pink grapefruit escalope recipe, peel 3 pink grapefruits and remove the white skin; cut them into rounds. Roast 4 tuna steaks of 150 g each in a large non-stick pan, without seasoning, for about 3 minutes per side. Add salt at the end, remove from the pan and keep warm. Pour the juice of a quarter of a grapefruit into the cooking liquid, add salt and cook until it has reduced by half. Turn off the heat and add 4 tablespoons of oil and the grapefruit slices. Serve the sliced tuna steaks with the grapefruit. Top with toasted breadcrumbs along with chopped pistachios and sesame seeds. Decorate with fresh chervil.

**BITES OF SALMON
IN THE SPECK WITH
SWEET AND SOUR
VEGETABLES**

Time 40 min + 1h rest

ingredients

4 people

600 g of trumpet courgettes

500 g of fresh salmon fillet

200 g of datterini cherry tomatoes

30 g of pine nuts

16 slices of speck

1 spring onion, sugar

apple cider vinegar, salt

extra virgin olive oil

Preparation

For the recipe for salmon morsels with speck and sweet and sour vegetables, peel the spring onion and cut it into slices. Wash the dates and cut them in half. Wash the courgettes, cut them into slices and brown in a pan over high heat with a drizzle of oil for 6-8 minutes, together with the datterini tomatoes, spring onion and pine nuts. Sprinkle with a couple of teaspoons of sugar and a good pinch of salt. Transfer all the well-roasted vegetables to a baking tray, sprinkle with 2-3 tablespoons of apple cider vinegar, close the tray with cling film and leave to rest for an hour. Remove the skin from the salmon and cut the fillet into 16 pieces weighing approximately 35 g; wrap in a slice of speck and brown quickly in a pan on all sides (it will take at least 8-10 minutes).

SWORDFISH ROLLS WITH PAPRIKA AND COURGETTE CREAM

Time 1h

ingredients

4 people

600 g 6 thin slices of swordfish

200 g of courgettes

150 g of grated pecorino

4 slices of bread

tomato concentrate

sweet paprika

chives, thyme, salt

extra virgin olive oil

Preparation

For the recipe for swordfish spoolies with paprika and courgette cream, peel the courgettes, cut them into slices and brown them put them in a pan over high heat with oil, 1 tablespoon of water, salt and a little thyme; when they are soft, blend the eggs. Collect the bread slices cut into pieces, 2-3 tablespoons of tomato paste, the pecorino cheese and a couple of teaspoons of paprika in a bowl and mix until you obtain a ball; divide it into 12 balls. Cut the swordfish slices in half lengthwise. Wrap the balls of mixture in the 12 slices of swordfish and close the spools with a string of chives (alternatively, use kitchen twine). Place the Rocchetti on a baking tray lined with baking paper and greased with oil, also grease the Rocchetti, salt only the fish and bake at 180°C for 15-20 minutes. Distribute the courgette sauce on the plates and arrange the swordfish rolls. Complete to taste with ground pepper and courgette flowers.

HERB OMELETE

Time 20 min

ingredients

6 people servings

12 eggs

200 g grated parmesan

150g of fresh cream

chives

mint

parsley

extra virgin olive oil

salt and pepper

Preparation

For the herb omelette recipe, mix the eggs just enough to mix the yolks and whites: by beating them for a long time they become crumbly and the consistency of the omelette loses its toughness. Add the parmesan, cream, salt, pepper and a nice bunch of coarsely chopped herbs. Pour the mixture into a large pan, over high heat, in a thin layer of hot oil. When a crust has formed, lower the heat, cover with the lid and finish cooking without turning it. Serve immediately or at room temperature. Stored in the refrigerator in an airtight container, it is also good the next day.

HONEY CHICKEN WITH CRISPY VEGETABLES WITH JUNIPER

Time 1h 10min

ingredients

4 people

1 kg of colored carrots

2 chicken thighs

2 chicken thighs

rosemary, juniper

dry white wine

Acacia's honey

sugar

apple cider vinegar

sunflower oil

extra virgin olive oil

salt and pepper

Preparation

For the honey chicken with crunchy juniper
vegetables recipe, place the chicken in a
baking dish with 6 sprigs of rosemary, 1
glass of wine and a pinch of salt. Seal with
cling film so that as little air as possible
enters and leave to rest for about 15 minutes.
This helps crisp the skin during cooking. Peel
the carrots, then cut them in half lengthwise.
Cut the tapered part into curls with a potato
peeler and the thicker part into sticks. Place
the ribbons in cold water with a few ice
cubes to make them curl a little. Bring a pan
of salted water to a boil; add 3 tablespoons of
apple cider vinegar, 1 tablespoon of juniper
berries, then the carrot

sticks and 2 tablespoons of sugar; cook for 5 minutes, then add the ribbons and cook for another 3 minutes. Drain them and, once cold, season them with a drizzle of extra virgin olive oil, salt and pepper. Brown the chicken in a pan coated with hot oil, then add the rosemary, bay leaf and 3 tablespoons of marinade, 1/2 glass of water and salt. Reduce the heat, turn the legs and thighs so that all sides get flavor, then cover and cook for at least 30 minutes. Turn them every now and then. At the end of cooking, remove the rosemary. pour 2 tablespoons of sunflower seed oil and 1 tablespoon of acacia honey, obtaining a sort of emulsion; brush the chicken with it on all sides, turn the pieces and brush them on the other side; return to high heat and brown for 4-6 minutes.

MACKEREL WITH ARUGULA WITH HERBS AND OLIVES PESTO

Time 1h

ingredients

4 people

90 g of olive pâté

40 g of cleaned Arugula

4 mackerel fish

2 eggs

extra virgin olive oil

Marjoram

salt

Preparation

For the mackerel recipe with Arugul and herb and olive pesto, hard-boil the eggs and cook them for 7 minutes after boiling. Cool, shell them, recover the yolks and pass them through a sieve, obtaining the mimosa. Clean and fillet the mackerel; remove all plugs. Blend the Arugul with 40 g of oil and pour into a saucepan with another 300 g of oil. Heat up to 60°C and immerse the mackerel fillets. Let them cook at a constant temperature for 10-15 minutes, then turn them off. Mix the olive pâté with 1 tablespoon of chopped fresh marjoram. Serve the fillets drained from the oil and salted, completing with the mimosa egg, olive pâté and a few fresh Arugul leaves.

CHICKEN AND AUBERGINES WITH SWEET AND SOUR COMPOTE

Time 1h

ingredients

6 people

1kg 1 chicken

14 ripe but firm apricots

2 aubergines

half a red onion

vinegar, garlic

extra virgin olive oil

sugar

salt and pepper

Preparation

For the chicken and aubergine with sweet and sour compote recipe, open the chicken in half and cook both sides on the grill, crushing them a little, for about 20-25 minutes per side. Cut the aubergines lengthwise into slices a couple of centimeters thick. Rub with garlic, season with salt and oil and roast on the grill for 4 minutes per side. Open 6 apricots and grill them for 2-3 minutes per side. Prepare a sweet and sour compote: chop the red onion and sauté it in 1 tablespoon of oil, add 8 diced apricots, 100 g of sugar, a splash of vinegar, a drop of water, salt and pepper and cook for 20 -25 minutes . Serve the chicken with the grilled aubergines and apricots with the compote.

COURGETTES FRITTERS AND RADISH SALAD

Time 1h 50min

ingredients

6 servings

200 g of flour

200 g of courgettes

150 g of milk

30 g of anchovy fillets in oil

10 g of breadcrumbs

5 g of brewer's yeast

20 courgette flowers

6 radishes, 1 white turnip

honey, lemon

fresh oregano

extra virgin olive oil

parsley

salt and pepper

Preparation

For the recipe for courgette fritters and radish salad, mix the flour with slightly warm milk, crumbled yeast and a pinch of salt, obtaining a very thick batter. Leave to rest covered until the volume doubles (about 1 hour). Wash the courgettes and grate them with a grater with large holes. Then mix them with the batter, also adding 16 flowers, cleaned and divided into strips.

Cook the mixture in a pan with 4 tablespoons of oil, pouring it into pancakes of about 10 cm in diameter. Cook them for about 2 minutes per side. Blend the breadcrumbs with 15 g of oil, the anchovies, 10 g of honey, 35 g of lemon juice, 40 g of water and a few parsley leaves with an immersion blender to obtain a sauce. Peel and slice the white turnip very thinly and cut the radishes in half. Add the remaining courgette flowers and season with oil, salt, pepper and fresh oregano. Serve the pancakes with the radish salad and sauce.

RAW COD

Time 25 min

ingredients

4 people

500 g desalted cod

400 g of mixed tomatoes

1 pink grapefruit

sugar

lemon thyme

fresh aromatic herbs

extra virgin olive oil

salt, black pepper

Preparation

Cut the cabbage into thin slices. Place them in a baking dish and season with a drizzle of oil, lemon thyme and black pepper. Let its flavor. Cut the cherry tomatoes into small pieces. Heat 3 tablespoons of oil in a pan with the lemon thyme. Sauté the tomatoes for 5-6 minutes, moving them without crushing them. Add a pinch of salt and 1/2 teaspoon of sugar. Finally, add the juice of 1/2 grapefruit and the pulp of the other half, taken with a spoon and broken into pieces. Plate the cod slices on cherry tomatoes and grapefruit, finishing with a drizzle of oil, pepper and fresh aromatic herbs.

CHICKEN BITES WITH LEMON AND GREEN PEPPER

Time 45 min

ingredients

4 servings

500 g of chicken breast

2 lemons, an onion

soy sauce, fresh ginger

sage, flour, dry white wine

salted capers, chervil, salt

extra virgin olive oil

dried green pepper

Preparation

Peel the onion and cut it into small pieces. Cook it gently in a saucepan for 5 minutes, with a drizzle of oil, 10 g of ginger cut into stripes and a sage leaf. Peel a lemon, divide it into wedges and peel them; Coarsely chop a spoonful of green peppercorns and desalt a spoonful of capers. Cut the chicken breast into bite-sized pieces and marinate it for 15 minutes with the juice of one lemon and two tablespoons of soy sauce. Drain the chicken and dry it with kitchen paper. Flour the chicken pieces and cook them in a large pan with a thin layer of oil for 5-6 minutes, then season with salt. Pour the pan where you cooked the chicken with a glass of wine for 3 minutes, then add the onion and chicken nuggets, mix well and cook for a minute. Serve the chicken, garnished with peeled lemon wedges, capers and a few chervil leaves.

BREADED CUTLETS AND MUSHROOM SALAD

Time 15 min

ingredients

4 servings

350 g 2 slices of veal sirloin

140 g of sliced champignons

50 g of flaked almonds

50 g of breadcrumbs

2 eggs, flour

fennel, lemon

Peanut oil

extra virgin olive oil

pepper, salt

Preparation

Mix the breadcrumbs with the flaked almonds. Dredge the steaks in the flour, shaking off the excess well, then in the beaten eggs, and finally in the breadcrumbs with the almonds, pressing a little to make it adhere well. Fry them in a pan that fits them properly, in plenty of peanut oil, for a couple of minutes on each side. Drain the steaks on kitchen paper, pat dry to remove excess oil. Blend a sprig of fennel with 3-4 tablespoons of extra virgin olive oil, salt, pepper, grated zest and the juice of half a lemon, obtaining an aromatic "green oil". Season the mushrooms with this oil and a pinch of salt and serve with the cutlets.

SWORDFISH WITH VEGETABLE SALAD

Time 30 min

ingredients

2 servings

2 slices of swordfish 1 cm thick

100 g of green beans

50 g of red onion

40 g of vinegar

10 red and yellow cherry tomatoes

5 passion fruit

extra virgin olive oil

salt and pepper

Preparation

Cook the swordfish slices in a pan with a drizzle of oil and a pinch of salt for 1-2 hours minutes per side. Remove it from the pan; dabbed with a sheet of kitchen paper, if you want to eliminate excess grease. Cut the onion into cubes and place it in a saucepan with the vinegar and 5 tablespoons of water. Let it simmer for 3 minutes after it comes to a boil; turn it off and let it cool. Peel the green beans and blanch them in boiling salted water for 4 minutes, cool in cold water and drain. Finally open them in half lengthwise. Cut the cherry tomatoes into wedges and remove the seeds. Open the passion fruit and collect the pulp in a small bowl. Blend with 2 tablespoons of oil and filter with a sieve to remove the seeds. Collect the green beans and cherry tomatoes in a bowl, then season them with a little passion fruit sauce. Serve the swordfish with a drizzle of oil and pepper and accompany it with the vegetables, the diced onion,

BAKED AUBERGINES

Time 2h 40min

ingredients

6 servings

3 aubergines

150 g of black olives

70 g of stale bread

50 g of cleaned salted anchovies

or anchovies in oil

50 g of salted capers

2 ripe tomatoes

a clove of garlic

extra virgin olive oil

dried oregano, parsley, salt

Preparation

For the baked aubergine recipe, peel and cut the aubergines in half lengthwise; cut the pulp into a grid, salt generously and let it rest for an hour with the pulp facing downwards. Chop a sprig of parsley. Chop the anchovies. Crumble the stale bread. Stone the olives. Desalt the capers. Chop the garlic. Blanch the tomatoes in boiling water for a few seconds, peel them, remove the seeds and cut them into cubes. Season the crumbled bread with parsley, garlic, capers, olives, anchovies, oregano and diced tomatoes. Mix well. Wash and dry the now purged aubergine halves; arrange them in a baking dish, and spread the aromatic bread and the second diced tomato on the surface. Season with oil and bake at 160°C for 60-70 minutes. Serve hot or warm, they are an excellent single dish.

CHICKEN WITH ERBS

Time 1h

ingredients

4 servings

1 kg chicken

125 g of whole yogurt

100 g of fresh goat's cheese

garlic, rosemary

tarragon, lemon balm

paprika, butter

extra virgin olive oil

pepper, salt

Preparation

Divide the chicken in half, cutting it along the spine, removing it and opening it like a book. Heat a few cloves of garlic

crushed with the peel, 2 sprigs of rosemary, a pinch of salt, a few leaves of tarragon and lemon balm, in a pan that can go in the oven with a knob of butter and 2 tablespoons of oil. Salt the chicken and season it with a teaspoon of paprika on the skin side, then add it to the hot herbs. Brown the first one on the skin side for 3-4 minutes, placing a weight on it so that it remains well pressed. Turn it over and cook it for another 2 minutes, then put it in the oven at 200°C for 30-35 minutes. Blend the yogurt with the fresh goat cheese, a pinch of salt, a teaspoon of oil and a little pepper. Serve this creamy sauce with the chicken.

**STEAMED COD
WITH AVOCADO AND
WATERMELON SAUCE**

Time 30 min

ingredients

4 people servings

600 g desalted and soaked cod

200 g of watermelon pulp

70 g of raspberries

25 g of almonds

1 avocado

watermelon and

raspberries for garnish

extra virgin olive oil

salt and pepper

Preparation

For the steamed cod with avocado and watermelon sauce recipe, blend the watermelon pulp with the raspberries, a pinch of salt and a little pepper. Filter to remove the seeds, then emulsify the smoothie with 2 tablespoons of oil. Cut the cabbage into slices and steam it for 7-8 minutes. Lightly toast the almonds in a pan and cut them into flakes with a knife. Peel the avocado and slice it. Distribute the watermelon and raspberry sauce onto plates and add the cod, avocado and almonds. Complete with watermelon, raspberry segments, a drizzle of oil and pepper.

**RED PRAWNS AND PEACH
AND RICOTTA SALAD**

Time 15 min

+ 1h of marination

ingredients

4 servings

12 pieces of red prawns

1 pc of ricotta

350 g of fine salt

Sugar (150g

3 peaches

fresh coriander

Lemon

extra virgin olive oil

Preparation

For the red shrimp and peach salad with ricotta recipe, mix salt and sugar; place the prawns, whole and in their shells, in a baking dish, cover them with the salt and sugar mixture and leave them to marinate for 1 hour. At the end, clean them from the marinade. Cut the peaches into chunks, and season them with the juice of 1/2 lemon, a drizzle of oil, a pinch of salt and a few coriander leaves. Arrange the scampi on a serving dish (you can shell the tails, for convenience) completing with the peaches and ricotta.

MACKERE FILLETS MARINATED IN LEMON AND SAGE OIL

Time 1h 20min

+ 1h of marinade

ingredients

4 people

850 g 8 mackerel fillets

300 g of extra virgin olive oil

250 g white asparagus tips

80 g of radicchio

2 untreated lemons

sage, salt

Preparation

For the recipe for mackerel fillets marinated in lemon oil and sage, clean the mackerel fillets, removing the belly part. Place them on the skin and cut them along the central bone, on both sides, up to the skin; fold the fillets slightly, so as to highlight the main bone, and cut it with scissors. Arrange the fillets in a baking dish. Season them with the grated zest of 1 lemon and the juice of 2 lemons and salt. Cover with cling film and let rest for 1 hour. Cut the asparagus tips into three slices each, lengthwise, and steam for 20 minutes. Heat the oil with a nice sprig of sage, bringing it to 140°C. Drain the fillets and discard the marinade; put them back in the pan and cover them with the hot oil. Let them rest until the oil has cooled. Fry the radicchio in a pan for 2 minutes with a drizzle of mackerel oil and a pinch of salt. Serve the mackerel with the radicchio and asparagus.

CHICKPEA BURGER AND ARTISAN KETCHUP

Time 1h 30min

ingredients

4 servings

For burgers

230 grams of potatoes

375 g of boiled chickpeas

2 egg yolks, sage, pepper, salt

extra virgin olive oil

For ketchup

250 g of tomato puree,

80 g of sugar

60 g of vinegar, salt

For the chips, 700 g of potatoes

extra virgin olive oil, salt

Preparation

Boil potatoes in their skins in unsalted water for 30-35 minutes after boiling. Drain them, peel them and mash them. Blend the chickpeas coarsely and then mix them with the potatoes, egg yolks, 5 chopped sage leaves, a spoonful of oil, salt and pepper. Form the mixture into 4 burgers, with a ring (7.5 diam.). Cook in a pan with a drizzle of oil for 15 minutes, turning them halfway through cooking. Prepare it while cooking the potatoes for the burgers: melt the sugar in a saucepan for 1-2 minutes, add the vinegar with the heat off, then turn on the heat to dissolve the lumps that have formed. Add the tomato puree and 50 g of water and cook for 8-10 minutes. Turn off the salt. Peel the potatoes, cut them into sticks, wash them in plenty of water to remove the starch, then dry them. Fry them in boiling oil for 5-6 minutes, drain them on kitchen paper and add salt. Serve with the burger and sauce.

ROAST LEG OF LAMB WITH ARTICHOKES

Time 2h 30min

ingredients

4 people

1.2 kg 2 legs of lamb

200 g of vegetable broth

4 artichokes

1 small onion

1 carrot, rosemary

sage, mint, pepper, cumin

garlic, flour

Lemon. White wine

salt and pepper

extra virgin olive oil

Preparation

For the roast leg of lamb with artichokes recipe, place the legs in a baking dish and sprinkle them with rosemary needles and sage leaves, salt, pepper, cumin, a few slices of chilli pepper and a drizzle of oil. Massage them above and below, then add 1 clove of garlic, the sliced onion, the peeled carrot slices, 1/2 glass of wine, and the vegetable broth. Bake the lamb at 180°C for 10-12 minutes, then cover it with aluminum foil and continue cooking for about 1 hour. Uncover it and cook it for another 1 hour. Blend the cooking liquid, filter it and then reduce it for about 10 minutes; add 1 tablespoon of flour mixed with 1 tablespoon of oil, to thicken the sauce a little. Clean the artichokes and cut them finely. Season them with oil, salt, lemon and mint and serve with the legs.

CHICKEN WITH LEMON AND NEW CARROTS IN PAPER

Time 35 min

ingredients

4 people

360 g 2 whole chicken breasts

4 new carrots

2 untreated lemons

coriander seeds

fresh coriander

extra virgin olive oil

salt

Pepper

Preparation

For the chicken with lemon and new carrots baked in foil, clean the chicken breasts from bones and connective tissue and divide them into two parts. Wash the lemons and cut them into slices. Peel the carrots and cut them into thin slices. Make small horizontal incisions on the breasts and insert the lemon slices. Transfer each breast onto a sheet of baking paper, together with the carrots; season with oil, salt, pepper and coriander seeds (press a little to release the aroma). Close the parcels and bake them at 180°C for 15-17 minutes. Remove the parcels from the oven, open them and top them with fresh coriander leaves and serve.

POTATO AND SPINACH MEATBALLS WITH LIME SAUCE

Time 1h 20min

ingredients

Portions of 50 pieces

650 g of spinach leaves

600 g of white pulp potatoes

80 g of breadcrumbs

60 g of pistachio flour

2 pieces of eggs

1 pc shallot

half a lime

wasabi paste, seed oil

extra virgin olive oil

salt fine and in flakes

Preparation

For the lime meatballs recipe, boil the whole potatoes in their skins for about 35 minutes; peel them, mash them and mix with the breadcrumbs, 1 egg and a pinch of salt. Chop the shallot and brown it in a pan with 2 tablespoons of extra virgin olive oil for a couple of minutes; add the chopped spinach and cook for 7-8 minutes; drain them from the cooking water, let them cool and mix with the potato mixture, keeping 20g aside. Form the mixture into round meatballs of 15 g each:

you will have about fifty. Dredge them in pistachio flour and fry them in plenty of hot seed oil for about 1 minute and 30 seconds; drain them on kitchen paper. Prepare a sauce by blending the reserved spinach with 1 egg, a pinch of salt, the juice of half a lime and 1 teaspoon of wasabi paste, slowly adding 130 g of seed oil. Season the meatballs with salt flakes and serve with the sauce.

SWORDFISH AND ASPARAGUS CARPACCIO WITH RASPBERRY SAUCE

Time 15 min

ingredients

4 servings

400 g of swordfish carpaccio

50 g of raspberries

40 g of hazelnuts

8 green asparagus

White wine vinegar

fresh coriander

salt

extra virgin olive oil

Preparation

For the swordfish and asparagus carpaccio recipe with raspberry sauce, blend the raspberries with 1 tablespoon of vinegar, 2 tablespoons of oil and a pinch of salt, obtaining a sauce. Peel the asparagus to remove the tough end part, peel the stems, then slice very finely, lengthwise, with a mandolin or potato peeler, so as to obtain ribbons. Arrange the swordfish carpaccio well spread out on the plates, arrange the asparagus ribbons, chopped hazelnuts, a few coriander leaves and drops of raspberry sauce on top.

EGGS IN A NEST OF LIME AGRETTI

Time 25 min

ingredients

4 servings

300 g of cleaned agretti

4 fresh organic eggs

White wine vinegar

black and white sesame

lime, salt

extra virgin olive oil

Preparation

For the lime nest egg recipe, bring a large pot of water to the boil with 4 tablespoons of vinegar (you will need it to cook the eggs). Boil the agretti in a pan of boiling salted water for 3-4 minutes.

Carefully crack an egg into a small bowl. Use very cold eggs from the refrigerator. Lower the heat under the pan and create a vortex by stirring with a spoon; pour an egg into the center by sliding it from the bowl; continue mixing very delicately to allow the egg white to envelop the yolk. After a few seconds, without removing the first egg, gradually repeat the same operations with the other eggs and cook them together for 3 minutes. The water should only tremble, never boil. Season the agretti with a drizzle of oil and a pinch of salt, available on the plates, forming small nests and place a poached egg in the centre. Complete with sesame seeds, a few segments and grated lime zest.

CHICKEN CACCIATORA WITH MARJORAM AND LIME

Time 1h 30 min

ingredients

6 people

6 chicken legs (free range chickens)

800 g of peeled tomatoes with their juice

1 red onion

1 clove of garlic

dry white wine

rosemary, marjoram

extra virgin olive oil

salt, pepper, lime

Preparation

For the chicken Cacciatore recipe with marjoram and lime, peel the onion and slice coarsely. Sauté it for 2 minutes in a large rondo with 3-4 tablespoons of oil, the garlic with its peel, a little rosemary and marjoram. Add the chicken legs and brown them over high heat for 7-8 minutes, browning well on both sides; season them with salt and pepper. Then blend with 1 glass of white wine, let it evaporate for 2 minutes, then add the juice of 1 lime. Crush the tomatoes with your hands in a bowl, so as to obtain a sort of very coarse puree, and add everything to the chicken. Lower the heat, cover with a slightly removed lid and cook for about 50 minutes. Check the cooking of the chicken from time to time and, if you see that the liquid has evaporated too much, add a little hot water. Complete with fresh marjoram, plenty of grated lime zest and garnish with rosemary flowers.

STUFFED ARTICHOKES

Time 1h 10min

ingredients

4 people

190 g of courgettes

60 g of fresh pecorino

20 g of spring onion

4 large artichokes

4 slices of bread

garlic, parsley

extra virgin olive oil

salt, pepper, lemon

Preparation

For the stuffed artichokes recipe, clean the artichokes by removing the tough outer leaves. Open them by digging inside to create space for the filling. Also keep part of the stems, peeled while keeping the heart. In a saucepan, bring 2 liters of water to the boil with 100 g of oil, a sprig of parsley, 2 slightly crushed garlic cloves with their peel and 1/2 lemon, lightly squeezed inside. Boil the artichokes by immersing them whole in this aromatic water for about 20 minutes. Drain them, place them upside down on a tray and let them cool. In the meantime, clean the courgettes and wash them.

Remove the crust from the bread slices,
blend in a cutter together with a handful of
parsley leaves and collect them in a bowl
with the grated pecorino and the green part
of the courgettes, grating until you reach the
central stone, where the seeds are. that you
can delete. Chop the hearts of the artichoke
stems and add them to the bowl. Chop the
spring onion and add it too, completing with
2 tablespoons of oil, salt and pepper. Mix
everything together to combine the filling.
Arrange the artichokes on a tray (positioned
at the four corners, so that they remain
closed and in shape more easily. If they tend
to open too much, tie them with kitchen
string). Fill them with the filling, grease them
with a drizzle of oil and bake them at 180°C
for about 10 minutes.

AUBERGINES CAKE

Time 1h 30 min

ingredients

4-6 servings

400 g of vegetable spreadable cheese

180 g of wholemeal croutons

150 g of cherry tomatoes

150 g natural tofu

10 pitted plums

2 streaked aubergines

coriander powder

cumin powder, peanut oil

extra virgin olive oil

pepper, salt, basil

Preparation

For the aubergine cake recipe, cut an aubergine into slices of a couple of centimetres, place them on a baking tray lined with baking paper and cook at 200°C for 25 minutes, then let them cool and add salt. Blend the wholemeal croutons with the plums and a pinch of salt. Blend the plain tofu and the vegetable cheese with half a teaspoon of ground cumin, half a teaspoon of ground coriander, a pinch of salt and a grind of pepper. Line a springform pan (20 cm in diameter) with baking paper and make the first layer with the croutons and chopped plums, flattening well until you obtain a compact base about half a centimeter thick.

Make a second layer with half the pureed tofu, then one with the aubergine slices and 50 g of cherry tomatoes cut in half. Cover with a final layer of tofu puree and bake at 180°C for 35-40 minutes, until the surface turns golden. Cook the remaining cherry tomatoes in a pan with a drizzle of extra virgin olive oil for a couple of minutes. Cut the other aubergine into very thin slices and fry them in plenty of peanut oil until they start to brown, then dry them with kitchen paper (aubergine chips). Decorate the cake with aubergine chips, pan-fried cherry tomatoes and a few basil leaves.

SWEET AND SOUR TURKEY CUBES AND FRUIT

Time 45 min

ingredients

Servings for 6-8 people

800 g diced turkey meat

500 g of new potatoes

12 fresh (or candied) cherries.

8 apricots

rosé wine, garlic

rosemary, mint

chopped pistachios

butter, salt

extra virgin olive oil

Preparation

For the recipe for sweet and sour turkey and fruit cubes, wash the potatoes and cut them very thin, rinse, blanch them in boiling salted water, drain and dry them. Brown in a knob of butter with a sprig of rosemary and 1 clove of garlic with the peel for a few minutes. Cut the apricots in half and brown in a pan with a knob of butter; when they start to caramelize, add 1 glass of passito wine and reduce the liquid until it obtains a syrupy consistency. Remove from the heat and add the cherries. Brown the turkey cubes in another hot pan with a thin layer of oil; finally glaze it with the apricot sauce and add the fruit. Serve it with potatoes, completed with mint leaves and pistachios.

SHRIMP POTATO AND LEEK CREAM AND MANDARIN REDUCTION

Time 1h 20min

ingredients

4 people

1 kg of mandarins

600 g of potatoes

500 g of leeks

20 prawns, chervil

extra virgin olive oil

balance, pepper

Preparation

For the prawns, cream of potatoes and leeks and mandarin reduction recipe, peel the potatoes and cut them into small pieces. Clean the leeks, eliminating the outermost sheaths, the final beard and the green part;

First cut it in half lengthwise and then slice it thinly. Cook the potatoes and leek in a pan with a couple of tablespoons of oil over high heat for a couple of minutes, season with salt and pepper; cover with water, then lower the heat and continue cooking for about 20 minutes, until the liquid has almost completely absorbed. Blend everything to obtain a cream. Peel the mandarins and extract the juice (you will get about 600 g). Simmer the mixture on the heat for at least 20-30 minutes, until you obtain a sauce with the consistency of syrup; remove from heat and sieve. Clean and shell the prawns; season them with oil and salt and drain them in a non-stick pan for 1 minute, then turn them over and cook for another minute. Distribute the potato and leek cream on the plates, place the prawns on top,

FILLETS OF GURNARD IN MUSTARD BUTTER

Time 40 min

ingredients

4 people servings

800 g of gurnard fish fillets

30 g of mustard

broth or fish stock

1 cucumber, 1 tomato

1 shallot, dry white wine

lemon, butter

chilli powder

extra virgin olive oil

salt and pepper

Preparation

To prepare the gurnard fillets with mustard butter, mix 75 g of soft butter with the mustard, the juice of 1/2 lemon and chilli pepper to taste. Peel the cucumber and cut it into 4-5 mm pieces. Blanch the tomato, peel it and cut it into cubes too. Blanch everything for less than 1 minute, drain and season with a drizzle of oil, salt and pepper. Massage the gurnard fillets with the mustard butter and leave them to rest in the fridge for 30 minutes. Chop the shallot and sauté it delicately with a knob of butter, blend with 1/2 glass of white wine, let it evaporate, then add 1 ladle of broth and reduce until you obtain a creamy sauce. Brown the gurnard fillets in another hot pan with the butter from the marinade. Serve them with the tomato and cucumber and season everything with the shallot sauce.

FISH THREE WAYS

Time 1h

ingredients

4 servings

1 kg char fish

clean and gutted

marten, Rosemary

parsley, lemon

remilled durum wheat

Grain semolina

vegetable broth

extra virgin olive oil

Peanut oil

salt, pepper, vinegar

Preparation

For fish, three ways: rinse the char and dry it. Cut it into three parts, just above the tail and just below the head. Stuff the central part with rosemary, marjoram and parsley, lemon slices, salt and pepper; grease the surface with a drizzle of extra virgin olive oil, then wrap the steak in baking paper and tie it like a roast with kitchen twine. Brown in a pan with a drizzle of extra virgin olive oil for about 3 minutes, turning it so that it browns all over the surface. Cook the roast in the oven at 180°C for about 20 minutes. Tie the head with a string or wrap it in cotton gauze, then tying it, in order to keep the pulp compact and in shape. Immerse LA in 2.5 liters of vegetable broth acidulated with 1 tablespoon of vinegar; let simmer gently for about 15 minutes. Flour the tail in the semolina and fry it by immersing it in plenty of not too hot peanut oil (160°C) for 6-8 minutes; drain it on kitchen paper. Reassemble the fish by combining the cooked parts in three different ways and serve it with sauces and lemon slices to taste.

FRIED ATLANTIC COD AND RADISHES WITH GREEN MAYONNAISE

Time 35 min

ingredients

4 servings

1 Atlantic cod fillet

250 g of mayonnaise

8 pieces briars, 3 eggs, milk

3 pickled green chillies

2 anchovies in oil

pickled capers

chopped parsley

flour, salt, soy sauce

breadcrumbs, peanut oil

Preparation

Peel the radishes and cut them in half. Beat the eggs with 10 g of milk and 1 tablespoon of soy sauce. Flour the cod fillet and dip it first in the beaten eggs and then in the breadcrumbs; repeat the operations a second time. Fry the cod in plenty of hot peanut oil for 6-8 minutes. Also dip the radishes in the flour, beaten eggs, and finally in the breadcrumbs and fry them in the peanut oil for 1 minute. Chop the green chili peppers, a handful of capers and the anchovies and mix them with the mayonnaise, adding 2 tablespoons of chopped parsley. Serve it with cod and radishes.

ROLLS, ARTICHOKES WITH MINT, AND CAULIFLOWER CREAM

Time 1h 20min

ingredients

4 people

700 g 12 thin slices of beef sirloin

500 g of cauliflower

12 slices of cheese

12 slices of bacon

4 artichokes, lemon

mint, seed oil

extra virgin olive oil

salt and pepper

Preparation

For the recipe for artichoke rolls with mint and cauliflower cream, clean the cauliflower and cut it into chunks; cook it in a pan with a couple of spoons of extra virgin olive oil over high heat for a couple of minutes, then cover with water, lower the heat, season with salt and pepper and continue cooking for another 20 minutes, until the liquid will not be almost completely absorbed. Blend until you obtain a cream. Clean the artichokes, cut them into slices and immerse them in water with a splash of lemon juice. Drain them and cook them in a pan with a drizzle of extra virgin olive oil for 4-5 minutes, season with salt and flavor with 3-4 chopped mint leaves. Add 1 glass of water and continue cooking for 7-8 minutes.

Season the beef slices with oil, salt and pepper; place a slice of bacon and one of the thin slices on the first quarter of each, then close by first folding the side flaps inwards and then rolling the slice to form a roll. Lightly salt the rolls and brown in a pan with a drizzle of extra virgin olive oil for 5 minutes; turn them and continue cooking for another 5 minutes. Transfer to the hot oven and finish cooking at 180°C for 7-8 minutes. Blend 30 g of mint leaves with 80 g of seed oil with a blender and heat at around 60 °C for 5 minutes. Sift it, let it cool and season the artichokes. Serve the rolls with cauliflower cream and mint artichokes.

**FRIED CHICKEN BITES
WITH SPICY GUACAMOLE**

Time 35 min

ingredients

4 servings

400 g of chicken breast

200 g of breadcrumbs

100 g of 00 flour

5 g of fresh coriander

3 files

2 ripe avocados

2 organic eggs

a fresh pepper

peanut oil, salt

Preparation

For the recipe for fried chicken nuggets with spicy guacamole, prepare the guacamole by cutting the avocado pulp into cubes. Add the juice of 2 limes, the finely chopped chilli and coriander and a pinch of salt. Cut the chicken breast into 3x3 cm cubes. Beat the eggs with a spoonful of water. Dip the chicken cubes in the flour, then dip them in the beaten eggs, finally dip them in the breadcrumbs. Fry the chicken in plenty of oil for 2-3 minutes, until it turns a nice golden colour. Salt the morsels and serve hot, garnished with lime slices and accompanied with guacamole.

**SALMON AND POTATOES
AROMATIC PAPER**

Time 1h

ingredients

4 servings

600 g of fresh salmon fillet

300 grams of potatoes

an egg yolk

a fennel

white vermouth

dill, mustard

lemon, peanut oil

extra virgin olive oil

pepper, salt

Preparation

For the salmon and potatoes in aromatic foil recipe, boil the potatoes for about 30 minutes, drain them, let them cool and cut them into slices at least 5 mm thick. Remove the skin from the salmon and check that there are no bones; if necessary, remove them with tweezers. Arrange the potato slices on a large sheet of baking paper, place the salmon steak on top and season with salt, pepper, a splash of vermouth, a drizzle of extra virgin olive oil and grated lemon zest; close in foil and bake at 230°C for about 15 minutes. Peel and slice the fennel very thinly, then immerse it in cold water for about ten minutes to curl it up and make it crunchy.

Finally, drain it and season it with extra virgin olive oil, salt and pepper. Prepare a mayonnaise by blending the egg yolk with a good teaspoon of mustard, the juice of half a lemon, a pinch of salt, and 100 g of peanut oil added slowly; finally add a generous sprig of chopped dill, mixing with a spoon. Remove the foil from the oven, arrange the potatoes and salmon on a serving platter, sprinkle with chopped dill and serve with the seasoned fennel and mayonnaise.

CONCLUSION

Dear reader, We come to the end of this exciting journey through the secrets of the Blue Zone diet of 2024. It has been an honor to guide you along this path to a healthier, longer and happier life. We hope that the information and advice shared on these pages has inspired and motivated you to make positive changes in your life. We would like to sincerely thank you for taking your time and attention to read our book. We hope you found the information useful and will apply it in your daily life to improve your overall health and well-being.

If you enjoyed the book and found what you learned useful, we kindly ask you to consider leaving a review. Your opinions are extremely important to us and other potential readers who may be interested in exploring the world of the Blue Zone diet. Thank you again for your support and for being part of this community dedicated to health and wellness. We wish you all the best on your journey to a life full of vitality, joy and longevity. With gratitude,

[KLARLOCK]

www.ingramcontent.com/pod-product-compliance
Lightning Source LLC
Chambersburg PA
CBHW051733250726
48659CB00001B/40